No One Ever Got Fat from Calories

--

The Real Truth Behind Weight Loss, Your Body, and Wellness

by: R. Belldon Colme

No One Ever Got Fat from Calories
The Real Truth Behind Weight Loss, Your Body, and Wellness

Published by Nutri-90 Wellness

Copyright © 2016 by R. Belldon Colme

ISBN-13: 978-1530786534

ISBN-10: 1530786533

Without Whom

For Imy and Devan,
without whose patience through my long and cranky days and
nights of writing, this book would never have been.

For Jason & Deborah,
without whose willingness to talk for hours about crazy details
this book would not make any sense to anyone.

And Holly,
Without whose editing skill and insightful contextual guidance
I would not appear anywhere near as polished as I do.

Thank you. I love you guys.

nutri - 90

Nutri-90 Books

nutri-90.com

Belldon Colme is a fifty-one-year-old life coach who believed his life was over due to heart failure in 2001. Having survived, he researched how the body works and discovered that tracking calories is misleading and that metabolism is central to healthy living.

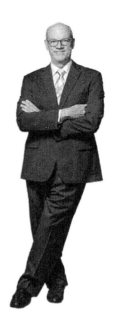

He developed a method to give the body's metabolism everything it needs to fulfill its role, and in 2004 he created Nutri-90, a wellness program that has helped thousands of medical professionals and laypeople alike reach—and maintain—their weight loss, health, and wellness goals.

R Belldon Colme

He currently lives in Redlands, California, with his loving partner Imy and their youngest son. He enjoys travel and adventure, but his passion is helping people reach a quality of life they never thought possible. Through Nutri-90, he provides personal wellness coaching, group training sessions, corporate workshops, and seminars to empower people to meet their wellness goals.

To learn more about personalized wellness programs and one-on-one coaching which will empower you to be the champion of your own life, including weight loss and cardiovascular and metabolic optimization, please visit:

nutri-90.com

{valuable coupons on back pages}

5

Contents

SECTION I

"There is only one cause of unhappiness: the false beliefs you have in your head, beliefs so widespread, so commonly held, that it never occurs to you to question them."

Anthony de Mello

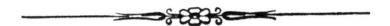

Chapter One
The End is the Beginning

I was completely disoriented; I could not understand why I was looking at cabinets from floor level. My thoughts were few yet overwhelming. Gradually, I became aware that I was on the floor and that these were the kitchen cabinets filling my vision. Someone was shouting at me, I sensed, but it was oddly silent, like a loud rock band on TV with the volume turned down. I had only two sensations: abject confusion and a growing realization that my pants were soaking wet.

Inexplicably, that latter thought began to frighten me. Had I peed my pants? Why were they so wet? Then a new thought hit me hard, even though I had no idea why or from where it had come: paramedics were on their way. I couldn't allow paramedics to see me if I had wet my pants. More fear. I pushed aside hands that were holding me down and sat upright. I stood and more hands accosted me, trying to steer me. I heard a voice I recognized but could not understand. Fear that I had peed my pants was my driving force for the moment, the one thing over which I felt I had any control, something I could solve. I stumbled to the bathroom to pee and change my pants.

Little bits of information began pushing into my consciousness, demanding attention, demanding clarity that I could not muster for them. My wife was saying something. My kids wore worried expressions. A knock sounded on the front door. Somehow I knew that was the paramedics. I clumsily tore off my pants and smelled them; the wetness did not smell like urine. It didn't really smell like anything at all. What was happening?

Wisp by wisp, the mental fog started to thin. I remembered I had been in the kitchen preparing coffee for the next morning. I remembered feeling... odd. Then, nothingness until the cabinets. My wife was saying something and I was finally starting to recognize the meanings of words. I told her I peed my pants, and please don't let the paramedics see me that way. She let out a weak chuckle through the lines of anxiety on her face and told me no, I had just dropped the coffee carafe on the floor when I fainted. I had water on my pants, that was all.

So I had fainted. That explained some things. A lot of fear vanished upon learning I had not peed my pants, but it was soon to be replaced by a different and more tangible fear: doom. Something grabbed my chest and began to crush everything inside. It wasn't anything I could see, but the force was devastating.

Paramedics hooked me up to wires from a small yellow box, strapped me to a gurney, and ran me to their van. As I was torn hastily from my home, a place I was struggling to recognize even though I knew I lived there, this new fear was shredding my consciousness. This was it. I didn't even get to say goodbye.

Chapter Two
The Wrong Recipe

Four times I have graced the emergency room for serious chest and heart problems. I am very fortunate to have never suffered an actual heart attack, although my symptoms have mimicked heart attacks so closely as to challenge disbelief.

The first ER visit was a wakeup call for me; my resting blood pressure two days after the incident was 170/105, a scary high number by any standard. I was advised by doctors and hospital staff that every risk factor of heart disease was elevated to alarming levels. I was 105 pounds overweight, wobbling on the edge of morbid obesity. On the day I was released from the hospital, I made the decision to make whatever changes were necessary in my lifestyle to regain my health, vitality, and well-being, whatever that would mean for me.

The late Dr. Stephen Covey, author of the renowned book, *The 7 Habits of Highly Effective People*, called this an emotion-based paradigm shift. Because of a strong emotional event, my deep-seated beliefs changed instantly, affecting my subsequent behavior. I often look back and wonder, *why*? Why did it take so much fear, and the belief that my death was imminent, for me to begin caring about my own health and well-being, to begin caring about my own survival?

In retrospect, the answer is simple: I didn't realize I was killing myself, how I was doing so, or why. Had you asked me back then, I would have bragged that I was a pretty good chef, a foodie even, and that I ate well. I laugh when I even type those words, because today I realize that my "recipes" amounted to:

1 box - powdery stuff
3 cans - wet stuff
½ pound - factory meat-like substance
1 bottle - gooey sauce

Mix together and heat until hot. Eat in front of TV while watching sporting event of choice

To greater or lesser degrees, that *is* a modern recipe. It is getting harder to find recipes that do not include at least one prepared, packaged food item. I understand now that I was not a foodie; I was a drug addict, legally addicted to the ever-increasing amounts of chemical additives placed in our groceries which manipulate us to buy a higher volume of lower-quality foods. "No one can eat just one" is more than a slick marketing campaign; it is the truth. Big Food, like Big Tobacco before it, is poisoning us with highly addictive additives that are both killing us and forcing us to almost helplessly buy more.[1]*

As I began to grasp these realities, I began also to change my eating habits. I read the books, sought my doctor's advice, and joined a popular diet plan. I diligently applied all that I learned, and I saw some level of success for my efforts.

And then I landed back in the ER. This time, my heart was beating violently and recklessly, fast and hard, as though it was being constricted by an inconceivable weight upon it and was struggling to free itself. I collapsed again, but this time remained conscious. All of my strength, it seemed, was being diverted to the epic battle in my chest. Once again, as I was

---

* Numbers refer to endnotes, located following the final chapter of this book. Symbols refer to footnotes, found at the bottom of the relevant page.

rushed to the hospital, I *knew* this was the end of everything for me.

Back home, having once more survived what had felt like imminent doom, I clearly remember sitting on the couch and feeling numb. As much as I tried to eat less and exercise and follow whatever other advice I could find, weight still seemed to creep up on me, and the scale was once again showing higher and higher numbers.

I was not the only one in my family afflicted with a frightening and serious disease. My father had recently died of a cancer his doctors said was largely caused by the food he was eating. My uncle had contracted the same cancer. Two of my sisters were to be stricken with different cancers, also affected by diet. It seemed my entire world was teetering on the edge of an abyss, and pushing me into that abyss was food, apparently the most sinister and deadly force in my life.

One day, mid-morning found me on the couch in my living room, still in my pajamas, desperate, depressed, and discouraged. A summer breeze was blowing through the open windows and there was a full mug of coffee in my hand. I was in a very strange head space, somewhere between blaming myself for my failures and trying frantically to figure out what to do, how to make things better and get myself healthy. As my thoughts all drifted together into that murky sludge where productive thought becomes impossible and dark becomes darker, a light broke through the gloom, an epiphany so bright that I realized in an instant what I had to do and what course my life would take from that point forward.

I had been trying everything to lose my excess weight, and I had been diligent. Nothing was working, but I realized in that moment that I was not alone. This stuff—the plans, pills, routines, systems, and programs—wasn't working for anyone. For every person I knew who had successfully lost weight, I knew 20 who were completely frustrated, body weight flying on and off like string thrashing wildly in the wind. I realized something with absolute certainty:

Something was not right with this process.

In that instant of time, a tsunami of bits and bytes of memory and information flooded my mind. I remembered my mom lecturing six-year-old me about eating my greens. I remembered church studies about balance. I remembered working on projects with my dad when I was young, my own business experiences as a home builder, words of my mentors, truths and lies I had experienced in the journey of my life. Yet I was able to piece them together and see, and that fact, the fact that I could intellectually see, brought something to the fore that changed everything. It was a relatively obscure bit of wisdom by a philosopher and mystic named Anthony de Mello:

"There is only one cause of unhappiness: the false beliefs you have in your head, beliefs so widespread, so commonly held, that it never occurs to you to question them."

I knew what I had to do if I ever hoped to heal and to become fit and healthy: I had to re-examine everything from a clear and open mind, a blank slate. What I learned in the ensuing process was nothing short of extraordinary.

In the pages of this book, you are going to learn truths so elegantly simple that they will resonate in every fiber of your body and soul, daring you to challenge them. But you won't, because they are true. Every biologist knows what you are about to learn. No chemist will dispute these words. Physicists recognize them as accurate. And yet, as de Mello so gracefully and eloquently observed, a lie has been sown in our minds, in the collective consciousness of our society, a lie so ubiquitous, so *everywhere*, that no one has ever thought to question it.

The Lie is the reason Americans spend more than $60 billion every year on weight loss, fitness, and wellness products and techniques, yet our obesity rates continue to climb with impunity.[2] It is the reason the last 30 years of our lives are overshadowed by chronic disease.[3] It is the reason two-thirds of us have difficulty enjoying the simple quality of life we so desire.

Understanding The Lie will open the door for you to also see The Truth. Applying what you are about to read to your own life will free you to accomplish some very important goals. You will finally be able to lose unwanted pounds, to be sure. More importantly, you will be able to keep those pounds from ever returning. More importantly still, you will understand how food and metabolism work and how that understanding leads to a much higher quality of life, largely freed from the so-called *diseases of civilization*. You will see that vitality, mobility, and a million of life's "little things" can finally be yours to enjoy every day.

SECTION II

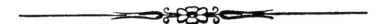

"Common sense is the knack of seeing things as they are, and doing things as they ought to be done."

C. E. Stowe

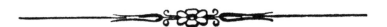

Chapter Three
The Beginnings of Common Sense

C. E. Stowe described common sense as "the knack of seeing things as they are, and doing things as they ought to be done." There is a simple yet extraordinary progression to this definition of common sense. It requires that we are first able to *see* things as they really and truly are before we can ever hope to *do* things as they ought to be done. You will not successfully drive a car with a standard transmission if you "see" it as an automatic. You will be very embarrassed at a formal black tie ball if you "see" it as a casual affair.

Prior to my light bulb realization, I had spent all of my time trying to do things as I believed they ought to be done: eating less and exercising to lose weight, taking my prescribed weight loss drugs, and trying the weight loss plans. I was trying desperately to balance my calories in and calories out. Yet I really had no idea at all *how things were*: how my body worked, how that weight got there in the first place. Nothing I was doing was working in any lasting way. Maybe, just maybe, I needed to step back and see things as they really are.

Once I directed my attention to seeing things as they are, doing things as they ought to be done came almost automatically. The actions I needed to take became self-evident. I am not saying it was always easy, but the who, what, where, and when became doable because I could plainly discern and understand the why and how of it all.

Believe me, the why and how is not at all what you might think it is.

In this section, you are going to learn three vitally important pieces of information. I am going to be very honest with you; when I made the decision to open my mind and discover nutrition through wide open eyes, I had to take a leap of faith. In order to find what would work for me, I had to accept that conventional diet wisdom might be fundamentally flawed. Maybe it worked for some, but it didn't work for me, and I am willing to bet it hasn't worked for you, either, at least not in the long term.

The truth, while simple and direct, is so far removed from what you have been led to believe that it is difficult to accept, even while it is impossible to deny. To accept the truth is to accept that you have been duped your entire life. It is to accept that you could have succeeded long ago and were held back by the greed and corruption of others. No one likes to admit having been conned, but it is important to accept it, get over it, and move on if you hope to see success now.

Moving forward, I ask you to take the same leap of faith that I did and, at least for the duration of these pages, allow your mind to be open and accepting of these new ideas. In this section, you will learn:

1. Metabolism does not "burn" anything at all. You will learn in simple and beautiful language what metabolism really does, and understanding it will change everything about how you perceive food and wellness.
2. Calories simply are not a factor in the human body. You will see that counting calories is making people chronically sick, and you will learn what you should be counting instead in order to be well. Once the blinder of calories is removed, you will clearly see the path to real and lasting weight loss.

3. The practice of treating parts of the body—metabolism, the heart, the muscular and skeletal systems, the kidneys, and the many other systems of the body—as separate entities is misdirected. Every part of the body is dependent upon the metabolism, and treating the metabolism treats every other body system simultaneously.

Remember, the goal of this section is to see things as they are. Once you clearly see things as they really and truly are, the next step, the doing step, becomes almost self-evident in its simplicity. That is the beauty of common sense.

Chapter Four
Why This Really, Really Matters

Let's set the stage for this conversation. "Calorie" is the most used word in the fields of nutrition, weight loss, and fitness, and even in many subcategories of health care. According to the experts, gurus, and even doctors, we are supposed to eat less of them, burn more of them, pay attention to where they come from, and so on. Ask any one of those folks what a calorie is, though, and the answer you get will be confusing at best, outright wrong at worst.

We will talk a lot more about calories in a later chapter, but for now I want to be very clear on something. Counting calories is making America sick. Very sick. The average American today spends the last 30 years of their life suffering from one or more chronic diseases and the last 10 years suffering major chronic disability. [4] These include heart disease, diabetes, kidney disease or failure, fatty liver disease, many forms of cancer, loss of mobility, and more. For many, those diseases come much, much sooner. All of that despite the fact that Americans spend more than $60 billion every year on products and programs based in calorie counting. If you hope to free yourself from this same eventuality, you must stop counting calories and start paying attention to nutrients instead.

To better understand, let's continue on to the second most-used word in the field of weight loss: metabolism. Seeing metabolism as it really is changed everything for me, and I bet it will for you, too.

In my workshops and trainings, I ask every room of attendees these three questions:
1. Who wants to be a little bit healthier?
2. Who wants to weigh less than they do today?
3. Who wants to *feel* better, more vital, and more energetic?

Not surprisingly, nearly everyone raises their hand to each of those questions. It is a stacked room, after all; guests are present for these very reasons. I then ask my attendees,

At the center of all three of those goals is the metabolism. Who can tell me what the metabolism actually does and how it does it?

If you do not know the answer, rest easy; you are in good company. I never see a single hand go up in response to that question. Few people know what metabolism is, let alone how it works. It is a mystery. All we are ever told about the metabolism is something like, "it burns calories and you need to boost it to burn calories faster."

But what if I told you that metabolism is the very reason life exists, and that without it there would be no life of any kind anywhere in the universe? What if I told you that your metabolism is the embodiment of every physical process that keeps you alive? What if I told you that even your emotional and spiritual strength depend on your metabolism?

Your understanding of metabolism is critically important. If metabolism actually were nothing more than an engine to burn calories and provide energy, then the equation we have been spoon-fed all of our lives would be true: less calories consumed and more calories burned would equate to sustainable weight loss.

But as you already know somewhere deep inside, *that equation can't be true*. Literally hundreds of millions of people put it to the test every year, and it has been estimated that the calories-in-calories-out (CICO) model fails them nearly 100 percent of the time;[5] they are rarely able to reach their goals, much less sustain them.

If, on the other hand, metabolism is much vaster in scope than you have been led to believe, if it is in charge of the

24

entire collection of processes that break down cells in your food and your body and rebuild their components into other, new cells that your body needs, we can recognize two things almost immediately:

1. The food you choose must contain something much different, something much more important than calories; it must contain all of the building blocks your metabolism needs to create all the various cells your body requires.
2. Since those new cells will be used for everything— replacing damaged or worn out tissues; growing new tissues like muscle, skin, and even brain tissue; creating immune system cells; and providing multiple forms of nourishment cells to keep it all working—your metabolism becomes responsible for not only your weight, but also your general health, vitality, longevity, and mental acuity.

Doesn't that give a new spin to what food is and how we should be using it? Food provides energy, sure, but it also provides every component the metabolism needs to literally build you, cell by cell. It follows that the quality of your structure can only reach the sum of the quality of those components, right? Basic chemistry dictates that something cannot be created from nothing. If you do not give your metabolism what it needs to build a certain required cell, that cell does not get built, or at least not properly.

The All-Important Number 90

Have you ever looked carefully at the nutrition label on a package of food? Featured right at the top of the label are numbers for serving size. Then there is a heavy black bar, under which there are numbers for calories, fats, carbohydrates, cholesterol, sodium, and protein. Then there is another heavy black bar, below which a few nutrients are listed.

This label is carefully designed for a deceitful purpose: the eye is naturally drawn between the heavy black lines, and folks don't really pay much attention to the numbers above or below them. We have been trained that if we see low-ish numbers between the bars, then we perceive the product as reasonably healthy.

But based on what you have just learned about the importance of your metabolism, that it builds all of the cells which keep your entire body in proper working order, the numbers at the bottom of the label become very important, because those nutrients are the very building blocks your metabolism uses to create that plethora of cells. It

Nutrition Facts

Serving Size 1/2 cup (115g)
Servings Per Container About 4

Amount Per Serving	
Calories 250	Calories from Fat 130

	% Daily Value*
Total Fat 14g	22%
Saturated Fat 9g	45%
Cholesterol 55mg	18%
Sodium 75mg	3%
Total Carbohydrate 26g	9%
Dietary Fiber 0g	0%
Sugars 26g	
Protein 4g	

Vitamin A 10%	Vitamin C 0%
Calcium 10%	Iron 0%

* Percent Daily Values are based on a 2,000 calorie diet.

TYPICAL NUTRITION LABEL
Images not otherwise credited are property of Nutri-90

follows that low numbers next to those nutrients are not okay at all.

On the label pictured here, there are four nutrients listed; vitamin A and calcium are present only in very low amounts, while vitamin C and iron are not actually present at all. Your metabolism requires so many more building blocks than these! Remember, what you get from your metabolism depends on what you provide it to work with.

Did you know *there are more than 90 nutrients required by your body to survive and thrive*? It is from this fact that my company derives its name, Nutri-90. For the curious, I have listed these 90+ nutrients in Appendix A in the back of this book. When you eat food, your metabolism breaks it down into its basic components—vitamins, minerals, amino acids, fatty acids, and other nutrients—and uses those components to build and maintain the varied cells and support the processes your body requires for health and vitality. *Your food must contain each of these 90+ components, and enough of each one*, for your metabolism to use in performing those tasks. There is no other viable source for these building blocks; if your food does not contain them, you become malnourished and your cell structures become weak and prone to illness.

The Processed Food Dilemma

Now here is the problem: modern food processing practices both strip food of its original nutrients and, at the same time, add chemicals, fillers, and *synthesized nutrients*, which actually inhibit absorption of nature-made nutrients by the body. Processed foods in general do not even pretend to have any meaningful nutrition, leaving the nutrition label blissfully blank. But even those processed foods that are "fortified" with essential nutrients fall woefully short because such nutrients are, by and large, factory synthesized; they are not recognized by your body and therefore are not properly absorbed.[6][7]

Take, for example, breakfast cereals and breads "fortified with iron." In order to prevent the added iron from changing the color and taste of cereal in unpleasant ways, the fortified iron is bonded to a chelating agent known as EDTA.[8] However, because EDTA is a chelating agent, that is to say a chemical whose primary medical purpose is removing heavy metals from the body when poisoning occurs, it actually prevents the absorption of essential metals and minerals that your metabolism needs.

Processed packaged foods are rife with such deceptive representations, making the food appear healthy while creating a nutritionally bankrupt product instead. As a result, the majority of Americans are malnourished, even though they have more than enough to eat.[9]

What Does It All Have to Do with Weight Loss, Your Body, and Wellness?

What we do not fully comprehend about the body and its myriad complex functions exponentially outweighs that which we do know. One thing we can proclaim with absolute certainty, however, is this: your metabolism is not a combustion engine. It does not burn, or incinerate, anything. Your body does not obtain energy, and certainly it does not acquire nutrition, from "burning calories."

What your metabolism does need to function is the full range of nutrients, the 90+ building blocks necessary to create every kind of cell essential to your body. To lose weight quickly, easily, and permanently, and to improve your health and well-being in the process, you must stop counting calories and start focusing on nutrition.

I know this idea flies in the face of everything you have ever been taught about weight loss and food. Do you remember earlier how I said that in order to learn about effective weight loss, I first had to accept the possibility that everything I thought I knew might be wrong? The insight I have just shared with you opened my eyes so much more than I ever could have imagined. This should be common knowledge, but for reasons we will explore as we go along it has been hidden from you, buried beneath layers of deception. I ask that you suspend doubt and disbelief just long enough to open-mindedly consider the rest of what you are about to learn. This will change everything about how you *see* your metabolism, and you will for the first time be empowered with successful mastery of food in your own body.

Chapter Five

The Secrets of Metabolism

It took me some time as a young man to understand what common sense is and how it works. We think of common sense as some inherent wisdom we are born with which instinctively serves us as we stumble through life, but that unfortunate understanding only limits the power of common sense to work in our behalf, adding to our personal oppression. It transfers our rightful power of self-direction to others by allowing them to define the words that govern our understanding of our environment. It limits our ability to "do things as they ought to be done."

As I said earlier, the brilliance of C. E. Stowe's observation is in the progression, for without the first part, "seeing things as they are," you can never effectively nor adequately comply with the latter part, "doing things as they ought to be done." Quite to the contrary; if you allow others to define "how things are," you can only become their pawns, acting in *their* best interests and working toward *their* ends rather than toward your own.

I frequently remind my coaching clients that *words mean things*. Your choice of words conveys much about the contents of your subconscious mind. Words you accept from others, together with the definitions you choose to accept for those words, program your subconscious, and from there your own thoughts and actions grow.

C. E. Stowe has told us why weight loss efforts fail over and over and over again: we have neglected to see things as they are before striking out and taking action. If you do not first see how things really are, how can you possibly expect to do things as they ought to be done? If you merely accept the words of others in defining how things really are, the best you can attain is to give them more of your hard earned money, hoping against all logic that this time it will finally work.

If the true answer to weight loss, improved health, and quality of life is the proverbial needle in the haystack, then the knack of seeing things as they really are is the magnet that will draw it out effortlessly. And once the needle is in your hand, the manner in which things ought to be done will become self-evident. From there, it will be up to you to choose the path you will follow for your own betterment and that of your family.

Metabolism is the most beautiful structure of processes and mechanisms in the universe, for without it there could be no life. But metabolism provides more than just a dull life, for without it there could be no sight to appreciate flowers and stars, no hearing to enjoy songbirds and thunderstorms, no taste or smell to bring joy to your nourishment. There would be no neural synapsis for thoughts and memories, no touch to appreciate the sensuous pleasure of our environment. We would have no means by which to recognize threats or opportunities. There would be no fear, no comfort, no pain, no ecstasy, no jubilation. There would be no consciousness, and therefore there would be only nothingness.

Metabolism is the reason living things exist and the means by which they function and thrive.

Inorganic matter is worn down by the environment until it is reduced to its most basic elements, then it becomes restructured by means of cataclysmic events: volcanos, collisions of tectonic plates, astronomical impacts, and earthquakes. Living things, by contrast, are constantly renewed and refreshed; cells are replaced, repaired, or fed in a never-ending chain of breaking down and building up of living cellular structures. This chain of events—this constant breaking down, rebuilding, and repair—is your metabolism. It is not a singular physical thing, nor is it a particular isolated process, but instead the combined processes that create and maintain life.

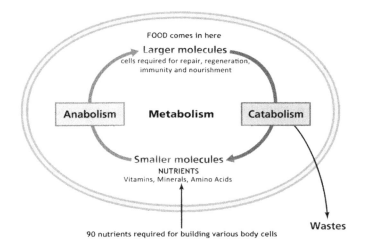

METABOLISM IS A NEVER-ENDING CYCLE OF MOLECULAR RESTRUCTURING.

In its simplest expression, metabolism consists of two main functions. *Catabolism* encompasses those processes that break things down in living bodies. These include digestion in all of its various forms, immune system eradication of foreign bodies, breakdown and removal of waste products, just for starters. *Anabolism* refers to those processes that build new living tissue and include healing of injuries; replacing and repairing worn cells; building trillions of new cells which allow children to grow and adults to be renewed; building immune antibodies to keep you healthy; and so on.

Everything metabolism does is accomplished within one of these two overarching categorical processes. Catabolism breaks things down, usually into their most basic pieces;

31

some become waste and others become raw materials for anabolism. Anabolism puts those raw materials together into the essential constructs your body needs to live and thrive.

Not long ago, I was outlining this process to a fourth grade class in one of my *Give Back* projects.[10] As I described how catabolism takes things apart and anabolism puts things together, an eager hand shot into the air and a smiling child exclaimed, "Like Legos!" Well yes, actually; exactly like that.[*]

A discussion ensued wherein we talked about Cat, a young girl who liked to take building blocks apart; and An, her friend who loved putting those building blocks back together again, creating wonderful and beautiful structures that each filled a useful purpose. Together, these girlfriends formed a club they called the Met Club.

In this story, which grew in richness and detail as we went along, Cat one day ran out of variety in building blocks to take apart. Suddenly, every structure she was given to take apart contained only red and yellow square blocks, all of the same size. When An saw the pile of blocks she now had to work with, she was dismayed; all she could build were simple structures that didn't perform their functional purpose very well, and which didn't look very pretty either. Still, the girls could only work with the blocks they were given, so they did their best.

Then a really terrible thing happened. Unexpectedly, Cat was given a different kind of structure to tear apart. The pieces were irregular in shape and they did not connect to the usual blocks the girls worked with. They literally fell apart for Cat, because they did not even connect to one another. An was

---

[*] Lego is a trademark of Lego Group. The views expressed in this book are not necessarily those of Lego Group or its affiliates.

not able to make anything at all with them, because nothing would connect with anything else. It was like working with building blocks from different manufacturers, blocks that were not compatible with one another.

Things became worse still for the girls when they began to receive things that were not building blocks at all. Cat was given sticks, stones, and broken pieces of unrecognizable garbage. These were not building materials at all! How could An possibly make anything useful from them?

Cat, of course, represents <u>cat</u>abolism. An is <u>an</u>abolism, and the Met Club symbolizes <u>met</u>abolism. This story was powerful to that fourth grade class, and I have used the same story many times since that inspired day, both with kids and adults. Here is how it works in your body.

When you eat a balanced diet of nutrient-dense real foods from nature, and by this I mean foods that come from the earth and have not been modified by factories, you are in effect giving your catabolism a wide variety of Legos to disassemble: thousands of blocks in all shapes, colors, sizes, and configurations, and all from the same set, as it were, designed to connect with one another to build useful and beautiful structures. Once catabolism has disassembled those blocks to their smallest pieces, your anabolism begins to build them into beautiful and useful structures for your body. Anabolism built your eyes, for instance, and your intricate ears, and even your heart that works tirelessly to transport your anabolism-built blood to every anabolism-built cell in your body. Anabolism quite literally constructed every single cell and structure that makes you *you*. And then anabolism uses the parts provided from catabolic activity to *maintain* your beautiful body in the very best manner possible.

When you choose foods with very few nutrients—for example, eating only breads and meats but no vegetables or fruits—it is like giving your metabolism only red and yellow square Legos. Your metabolism becomes very limited in what it can create to make and keep you healthy. Catabolism will disassemble them, and anabolism will do its very best to give you whatever measure of health it can, but the raw materials simply aren't sufficient to properly create and maintain what your body needs.

When you choose to eat processed foods with useless, nutritionally bankrupt fillers, it is like adding in building blocks from a different manufacturer; the pieces do not fit together, and all your catabolism can do is pass the useless filler off as waste.

Worst of all, when you choose to put "phood" into your body, meaning stuff we eat that is filled with toxic chemicals and mysterious ingredients that do not belong in a human body at all, it is like giving your metabolism sticks, stones, and broken pieces of unidentifiable garbage. Anabolism cannot connect the pieces provided and cannot adequately care for the needs of your body. Sickness is sure to follow.

I want you to remember this perfect analogy of building blocks, as we will come back to it again. Let's take a moment, though, to better understand each of the two categorical processes of metabolism. Remember, "Common sense is the knack of [first] seeing things as they are, and [then] doing things as they ought to be done." Only by understanding how things are, that is to say how things are working in your metabolism, can you then hope to do things properly to achieve your goal of weight loss and improved health and vitality.

How Metabolism Works

Let's get an overview of the greater processes by which food is broken down and repurposed in your body. That is what is going on, after all; in the same manner that a construction developer might tear down an old building and salvage bricks, antique fixtures, and old weathered beams and boards for use in new construction, your body is tearing down the food you eat and repurposing its usable components for new building projects inside your body.

Cat

When you eat food, catabolism breaks it down. This process starts immediately when you put food in your mouth and begin chewing. Chewing is a mechanical form of catabolism, and it starts the process of breaking food into smaller pieces. When you swallow, your food travels to your stomach, where it is subjected to chemical catabolism: a bath in hydrochloric acid. This breaks food down further and continues the process of transforming it into usable components for your body.

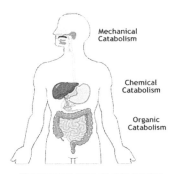

DIGESTION IS PART OF CATABOLISM
REPRODUCED BY PERMISSION FROM SCIENCE LEARNING HUB (THE UNIVERSITY OF WAIKATO). ©2007-2016.

When food leaves your stomach and enters the intestines, it is fermented by colonies of essential bacteria and enzymes— the flora and fauna, if you will, of your intestinal landscape. Here food is broken down into its smallest components, the individual Lego pieces, and the process of anabolism begins.

This description is oversimplified, to be sure, but it does outline the basic overview of how food is processed in your body: mechanically, chemically, and through fermentation. In fermentation, your foods are broken down into the smallest nutrient particulates, able to be absorbed into the bloodstream through the intestinal walls. Anything deemed unusable is identified here as waste and sent on through your body for excretion.

Notice that nowhere in the process of digestion, the catabolization of food, is anything incinerated. Nothing is "burned."

Remember, your goal is to see things as they really are, and in this process of discovery it is important to understand that words mean things. The phrases you use to describe metabolic processes will affect your decisions about the products you will allow into your body under the guise of food, drink, and even medicine. Make a note of this point, because we will come back to it in a bit.

Besides the breakdown of food, catabolism also encompasses the breakdown of any complex molecules in living organisms to form simpler ones. It is the destructive side of metabolism. If you damage muscle tissue during strenuous activity, catabolism will break down the damaged tissue for reuse or removal. If a foreign substance is detected in your body, your immune system hunts it down and captures it, and then catabolism breaks it down for elimination. Catabolism receives and breaks down the waste products from every individual cell in your body for removal via the bloodstream. Whenever something needs to be broken down, either for removal as wastes or to be repurposed by anabolism, catabolism is charged with the task, and performs it beautifully and efficiently.

An

The counterpart of destruction is rebuilding. Anabolism is the yin to catabolism's yang. As catabolism breaks down the food you eat and certain structures in the body required for maintenance operations, anabolism reuses those parts and pieces as needed in the process of building new cells and maintaining existing cells throughout your body. Much like a child will connect individual toy building blocks to create more complex structures, anabolism uses simple, small molecules to build larger, more complex molecules.

Anabolism is a truly incredible function, encompassing the ability to synthesize almost anything needed by your body, provided it has the basic ingredients—the building blocks—it needs.

Thanks to misleading marketing practices and the propensity of the American medical establishment to accept Acts of Congress as medical fact, we institutionally tend to believe that the things we eat go straight to our bloodstream and body cells. In most cases, nothing could be further from the truth. The things you eat generally do not enter your body in usable form. Catabolism must break them down into their most basic molecules, and anabolism must repurpose those basic molecules to build structures usable by your body.

Let's put anabolism and catabolism together and see what your metabolism is really doing in your body. Let's see what the Legos really are and why they are so very important.

The Met Club

Real food provides everything your body needs to thrive, but not necessarily in a form your body uses. For example, when we eat protein, it is not likely configured with the same set and distribution of amino acids we need for our own biological design. This is where we can best use the Lego analysis to understand the function of catabolism and anabolism, collectively known as your metabolism.

When you eat protein, extending the example, it is not passed on to your body in the form of the protein you ate. Instead, catabolism breaks it down into its smaller component parts: amino acids. There are 20 amino acids used by your anabolism in creating the various proteins you need. Amazingly, your anabolism can create 11 of those on its own so long as the Legos, that is to say the required nutrient parts and pieces, are available to do so. The remaining 9 amino acids are often referred to as *essential amino acids* because they must come from the food you eat.

Once your catabolism has broken all of your ingested proteins down into amino acids and anabolism has created the amino acids within its capability, your anabolism then connects the amino acid blocks back together into the many varied proteins needed in your body. Proteins are the workers in your body, performing everything from messenger services to taxi services and providing you the ability to move. Some protect your DNA sequences and control when and how your DNA is read. Proteins in mass coordination cause your muscles to expand or contract, facilitating your movement. Different proteins wrap themselves around other molecules, such as cholesterol, allowing their passage through your body.[11]

There are well over 100,000 different types and configurations of proteins present in your body; some researchers believe there are 2 million or more.[12] Yet none of this plethora of proteins come directly from the proteins you eat. All of them are created by anabolism from the amino acid building blocks that become available after catabolism disassembles eaten proteins into their smallest usable pieces.

This same breakdown/buildup process is used by your metabolism for nearly all of the foods you eat. Almost nothing passes directly from your food to your body for immediate use; instead, it is all broken down by your catabolism into its smallest building blocks and then rebuilt by your anabolism into whatever your body needs.

Macro-molecules	After Catabolism	Anabolism Makes
animal proteins plant proteins	amino acids	proteins used by your body
animal fats plant fats	fatty acids	fats used by your body
carbohydrates (carbs)	sugars	glucose and parts for ATP molecule
nucleic acids	nucleotides	DNA and RNA
remaining parts of food	vitamins, minerals and other nutrients	everything your body requires

You may have heard the term "macronutrients." This moniker is somewhat of a misnomer, because these are not actually nutrients in and of themselves at all. We will instead call these "macro-molecules," because the protein, fat, carbohydrate, and nucleic acids we eat are large molecules that our anabolism breaks down into smaller molecules, and these smaller molecules are the actual nutrients your anabolism then uses to build the larger molecules your body really requires.

A notable fact about the catabolic/anabolic cycle is that anabolism builds only what is necessary for your body to function and thrive. Leftover building blocks, those not required, are eliminated from your body as waste.

That is a powerful fact. This is where folks want to stop me and ask, "Then why do we get fat? If the body throws out what it doesn't need, why do we get fat? If fat we eat does not become body fat, why do we get fat?"

That is a great question and I will answer it, I promise. Before the answer can be understood, though, we have to continue a bit more with this process of seeing things as they are. Along with understanding what your metabolism is really doing, you also need to understand what a calorie is—and isn't—and its place in nutrition science.

Chapter Six
Calories—The Science and History

There is a great deal of misinformation in the world. Some of it is based on bad knowledge but good intention. Some of it is based on purposeful manipulation. Still more of it is based on ideas that were once widely believed but have since been proven wrong. The most insidious misinformation, though, is based on corporate profit, and corporations are often willing to sacrifice the well-being of individuals like you and me in order to squeeze a few more dollars into the next quarterly report.

Do you remember my earlier quote from Anthony de Mello? "There is only one cause of unhappiness: the false beliefs you have in your head, beliefs so widespread, so commonly held, that it never occurs to you to question them." In my experience this is true, and calories are no exception. Nearly 60 percent of the U.S. population is seriously overweight, a number that is growing fast. Obesity has reached the point where the United States has officially listed it as a disability and created a protected status for it.[13] As established earlier in this book, the average American spends the last three decades of his or her life, 30 years or more, chronically ill, unable to enjoy their life fully and sometimes unable to enjoy it at all. All of this has led to much unhappiness, and that unhappiness can all be traced to one false belief, a belief so widespread, so commonly held, that it never occurs to anyone to question it. You see, *there is no such thing as a calorie in your body*. In fact, a calorie is not a physical thing at all. It could not be burned even if you wanted to do so.

Let's talk about calories for a bit and you will understand why I can make such an assertion. Read this section with an open mind and let it run through your own sense of reason. In my experience, people find the truth about calories very hard to believe, even though they see the factual nature of it right away. We as a society are simply too invested—emotionally, morally, financially—in the propaganda we have been fed about calories. Recognizing that it has all been a farce is a hard pill to swallow, but doing so will free you in ways you may not yet imagine. In particular, it will free you for a lifetime of health, vitality, and quality of life.

Science

The definition of a calorie is simple.

calorie - unit of measure of the heat energy needed to raise the temperature of 1 gram of water through 1°C

In nutrition a slightly different definition is employed, the two being technically differentiated by the capitalization of the letter C:

Calorie - unit of measure of the heat energy needed to raise the temperature of 1 kilogram of water through 1°C (also known as a Kcal or a kilocalorie)

In other words, when talking about food we are talking about thousands of calories. That means your Whopper, listed as 660 Calories (big C) when incinerated (literally burned), actually releases 660,000 calories (little c) of heat energy. That is enough heat to raise the temperature of a bathtub of water more than 10°F!

From this point forward we will use the lower case "c," "calorie," for our purposes, unless we are listing the caloric value of a substance or referencing a specific source. To avoid confusion just remember, 1 Calorie (big C) equals 1,000 calories (little c).

The important thing to note here is that a calorie is not in and of itself a physical thing. A calorie is a **unit of measure**, nothing more and nothing less. As a unit of measure, it cannot be burned. It cannot be held. It cannot be stored. Like an inch or a gallon, it can only measure something else: increased heat, in this case.

In my workshops, I hold up a box and explain to my guests that I collect inches. I use what inches I want or need, and I store my leftover inches in that box to use later. Sometimes I run into a problem when I collect too many inches, and I find I need to make a bigger box! I even offer, because I am a thoughtful guy, to share my inches with anyone in my audience who may need more inches than they have.

Can you imagine the looks on the faces of my guests? Those looks are priceless; everyone looks at me incredulously. Everyone knows that an inch is only a unit of measure, used to determine how long some other thing is; inches cannot be collected, shared, or stored. Inches are not a physical thing.

But you see, calories, like inches, are also only a unit of measure, and are not a physical thing.

And since calories are not physical objects and they are not energy—only a *unit of measure* of heat energy—they cannot be eaten, burned, stored, or otherwise utilized in any way. This, in turn, means we have all been subjected to a false belief. We have been told that if we eat less calories than we burn, we will lose weight. But how can that be if calories are not an object that can be eaten or burned? How can that be if, as you learned in the previous chapter, metabolism does not burn anything at all?

Remember how I keep saying that words mean things? *Definitions* of words mean things, too. If words are used to describe nutrition that ignore the definition of calorie, words that fly in the face of what a calorie really is, one can only become confused. And indeed we have.

The calories-in-calories-out (CICO) model for bodily energy balance does not work, and it never has. Rather than abandoning it, though, the experts try to "explain it better."

When was the last time you heard someone exclaim that "not all calories are the same"? Probably today or yesterday, and certainly recently. They are trying to justify the fact that weight loss happens with some foods and not with other foods, even though the calories listed may be similar. But all calories *are* the same. Exactly the same. A calorie is a measure of the rise in temperature when something is burned. The definition never changes. Ever. Saying that not all calories are the same exacerbates a false belief. Wouldn't it be better to eliminate the calorie from the statement and simply say, "Not all foods are the same"? That, at least, would be true.

In order for a calorie to exist, there must be four things: a fuel, a source of ignition, water (or similar liquid with consistent properties when heated), and a thermometer. The fuel is incinerated completely until all that is left is black carbon. The heat released from that incineration is absorbed by water surrounding the burning sample. The resultant rise in water temperature is then measured to determine how many calories of heat were released by the fuel.

In order for a calorie to be a thing in your body, then, your metabolism would have to incinerate your food until all that was left was black carbon, and you would measure the resultant rise in temperature of your body liquids surrounding the incineration process. Only then would a calorie be a consideration in metabolic function. Of course, you would then suffer body temperature changes of tremendous proportions (remember how an incinerated Whopper could raise the temperature of 30 gallons of water more than 10°F?). You would also poop briquettes, and that would hurt.

Obviously this is just silly. In his book *The Fallacy of the Calorie*, Dr. Michael S. Fenster, MD, puts it this way: "There are not many absolutes when it comes to human physiology. However, you absolutely do not process food by turning it all to ash and naught."

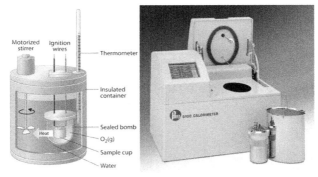

MODERN BOMB CALORIMETER WITH INTERNAL NOMENCLATURE
Photo credits: Averill, Eldredge, General Chemistry: Principles, Patterns, and Applications, v. 1.0 (Parr instrument Company)

Some still defend the calorie by asserting it does not mean the same thing in nutrition science, that it is actually a statement of the energy value of foods and is calculated differently than in other scientific fields. But is it, in fact, 'calculated differently'? No. In calculating the caloric energy value of foods, regulatory agencies burn them down to carbon and measure the rise in temperature of surrounding water. This is done using a device called a *bomb calorimeter*, depicted above.

To be completely factual, today's food manufacturers use a printed table to determine the caloric values placed on food labels. The chart lists the caloric values to be used for proteins, fats, and carbohydrates. A food manufacturer then determines how much protein is in the food, how much carbohydrate, and so on, and adds up the calorie figures from the table. However, the caloric values on that table were all determined using the bomb calorimeter.

As you can see from the diagram on page 45, all calories are indeed the same, and they are all calculated using an archaic method that simply is not applicable to nutrition and the human body.

You might reasonably ask, "How, then, did it come about that calories are an element of modern nutrition science?" And that is an awesome question. To answer it, let's depart from science for a moment and take a look at history.

History

"Calorie" was first coined as a word in the early 1800s by French scientists working on the efficiency of steam engines.[14] In this context, it made a lot of sense to work with a unit of energy defined as the extent to which a burning fuel raises the temperature of water; that is exactly what one wants a fuel to do in order to create the steam that runs the engine. There was a basic flaw in the term, though. "Calorie" was derived from the French word *caloric*, believed to be a fluid that embodied heat. In other words, researchers at the time mistakenly believed *caloric* was a *substance* in fuel that was responsible for the heat output when it was burned, and calories were a means to measure how much of the (non-existent) substance a given fuel contained. [15] We later learned that there is no such thing as the physical substance caloric, yet the underlying notion has persisted, along with the word calorie.

It was a chemist, William O. Atwater, who cemented the word calorie into the study of human nutrition in the late 1800s. Atwater was tasked by the US government with determining how to feed workers to deliver the most work output for the least expensive food input. He faced a few serious challenges in completing that task. How would he quantify the energy content of food? How would he quantify the energy output required for completion of various work tasks? With the very limited understanding of metabolism available to him at the time, Atwater went to work.

There was only one word in the English language used to quantify energy in the late 1800s and that was calorie, and so it was that Atwater used the unit in his research. However, he used a bit of creative math in order to make his research reasonable. Steam engines had an efficiency rating of about 10 percent, meaning about 90 percent of the energy derived from the fuel source was lost through the works and only 10 percent actually pushed the train. Atwater determined that humans and animals functioned at between 20 and 30 percent efficiency.[16] His observations and subsequent math were based on that idea.

I want you to realize at this juncture that all sciences have long since relinquished use of the word calorie as a unit of energy. Calorie is a unit of heat released by incineration of a substance. Each science has since created vocabulary and equations to more directly define specific forms of energy, be it chemical energy, light energy, electrical energy, mechanical energy, and so on. Only nutrition science holds on to this archaic and misused unit of measure. While it can be (and is) argued that all forms of energy can be mathematically interchanged, we will see in a few pages why the math does not add up when discussing food in the human body.

Atwater completed his work under direction of the U.S. Food and Drug Administration (FDA) in the late 1800s and very early 1900s. His calculations stand in the FDA to this day, and are referred to in FDA food labeling guidelines as *specific Atwater factors*.[17]

Now for the historical rub. What we know today about metabolism through research in the sciences of micro-biology, cellular biology, modern chemistry, physics, and other sciences began to emerge in the mid-1900s, long after Atwater's research was completed. As early as the 1920s, it was suggested that the FDA choose a different unit of measure for food and nutrition sciences. The FDA elected to maintain the status quo, though, arguing that the American public was already used to calories in nutrition and would have too difficult a time adjusting to the change.[18]

Today, while specific understanding of the minute details of energy workings in the body are still elusive, we nevertheless have a much greater knowledge of how metabolism works and how energy is actually distributed and used in the body. Even so, we are still striving to shove the old square peg into our modern round hole by applying ever more complicated math to equations that simply will not balance.

Scientifically, "calorie" is a misleading and inaccurate measure of the value of food in the body. Historically, the calorie in nutrition should have died together with the calorie in every other science. Even for heat, scientists now use the unit *joule*, while engineers often use *British thermal units* (BTUs), both of which are direct expressions of heat, and do not require the intermediary of water. It is only by an act of the FDA that the calorie is still being used in nutrition, and the very basis for its use started with a lack of any other available English word coupled with an inaccurate belief that it was measuring an actual liquid substance.

One last note before we leave the history behind. Atwater's work was not designed to determine how to keep a human being healthy or in optimum condition; it was designed only to get the most work from the least expensive food. Remember that, because the basis has not changed much in all these intervening years. Today's giant corporations are largely interested in providing the most "energy" from the cheapest materials, too. It is also worth noting that Atwater was known for his wide girth, as he was substantially overweight himself; he was not researching health and wellness.[19]

Chapter Seven
The Only Three Things You Need to Know About Food & Your Body

Here's the thing: energy management is only one small part of the role of metabolism, and providing an energy fuel is but one small part of the purpose of food. Let's take a look at three important facts about how food is used in your body. This chapter will begin to open the door to an understanding of exactly how you can take charge of your metabolic health, including weight loss, cardio-vascular optimization, and total body health. In other words, this chapter will help you learn how to take charge of your wellness.

Fact #1 - Food is Your Body's Lego Set

While scientists incinerate every particle of a food until there is nothing left but a pile of carbon to determine its caloric value, in your body as much as 20 percent of your food is almost immediately eliminated as waste. When digestion is complete, there is a mass remaining that is simply eliminated, entirely unused.

Of that portion of your food that is digested, most of it is utilized in body maintenance. Remember the Legos? Your food delivers the building blocks to your body.

The protein you ingest is broken down into its basic blocks, the 20 amino acids your body needs in order to synthesize its own necessary proteins. The proteins in your body are being repaired and replaced in a constant cycle, requiring a constant influx of protein from your food. Of the 20 amino acids your body requires to carry out this task, 11 can be synthesized by your body itself, but 9 cannot and must come from food sources. Incinerated amino acids would be useless to your body in this process, right? Although proteins are considered calories on food labels, the truth is that your body does not utilize many proteins as fuel, using them instead as blocks to build, repair, and maintain cell structure; communicate important messages throughout each body system; and taxi other particles through the bloodstream to name just a few of its multitude of functions.

Fats are similarly misunderstood. Clever advocates of the food industry teach us that fats eaten are converted to fat in the body, unless of course we "burn" those fat calories first. Food labels assign fats a caloric value, different than the value attached to protein. Fats, though, just like proteins, are broken down into their smaller particles through digestion, fatty acids, and repurposed in your body. Fatty acids are used in your body for everything from building cell wall structures to acting as fat-soluble vitamin carriers. Fatty acids can be further broken down to facilitate inflammation (important for calling immune system help to an injured site) and de-inflammation, local area hormone structures, and blood thinners just for starters.

Ingested DNA and RNA, or more specifically nucleic acids, are broken down into nucleotides that will be restructured into nucleic acid molecules consistent with human makeup.

Carbohydrates, which you likely refer to simply as *carbs*, are broken down into sugars, the most common one in your body being glucose.

These four groups—proteins, fats, carbs, and nucleic acids—are known as macro-molecules and they compose four of the basic groups from which nutrients are extracted in the body. Think of these as the Lego sets that catabolism is given to start with. They are the first things in your food that are identified by your body and broken down into their substructures by means of catabolization.

In a perfect world, your food comes primarily from plants and other animals and, as such, the protein, fat, carb, and nucleic acid macro-molecules from your food sources are not configured in the form needed by your human body. Hence catabolism breaks those Lego sets down into their individual Lego pieces, and anabolism restructures them into the macro-molecules required by your body.

There is much more to your food than these four macro-molecules. Some assert that there are just 11 vitamins and 4 minerals essential to good health, but there are, in fact, more than 90 essential nutrients that your body needs to survive and thrive.

You can easily discern already that nothing at all is in any way "burned" in these processes, right? If the food you ate were burned up as energy, where would the necessary Legos for building the cells in your body come from? On the contrary, the catabolized Legos are needed in their whole, unburnt state in order to be useful for building, repairing, and maintaining your body.

It follows that the *majority* of the food you eat is repurposed by your body according to its needs. This is perhaps the most important piece of information about your metabolism that I can impart to you, because it illustrates what you truly must focus on if you are to achieve a measure of health and wellness: you need to focus on the quality and type of Lego sets you choose to provide for your metabolism. You need to stop focusing on calories, which are not even things in your metabolism, and focus instead on the *nutrient* quality of your food, because those nutrients are the Legos, the building blocks, that your body is using to make and keep itself fit and healthy. Those nutrients are involved in every aspect of your existence, from physical structures to spiritual awareness to mental acuity to emotional well-being.

It is time: STOP counting calories and START paying heed to your Legos, the nutrient content of your food.

Fact #2 - Yes, Food Does Provide Energy for Your Body

Yes, your body uses energy. It does not come from heat like a steam engine, however. It comes from a chemical reaction involving a molecule often referred to as the "high energy molecule": adenosine triphosphate, or ATP for short. We call ATP the energy currency of the body, and it exists in every cell of your body for use whenever energy is required.

ATP releases energy when a chemical bond between its phosphate groups is broken. Whenever energy is needed— by a process, a protein, or even by anabolism itself—a phosphate bond is broken in the ATP molecule, providing the needed energy. ATP is thus catabolized, or reduced, to a smaller molecule: adenosine diphosphate, or ADP.

Now that the required energy has been delivered, ADP needs to be recharged, like you might recharge a battery, before it can be used as an energy source again. This recharging is done inside each cell by the mitochondria, which receive the ADP molecule and add another phosphate group via anabolism, turning it back into ATP. The ATP is then ready to provide energy again whenever needed. This process of ATP becoming ADP and then being recharged back into ATP is known as *cellular respiration*.

Cellular respiration utilizes Legos from our food. Glucose is the primary ingredient, making carbs an important part of our daily eating plan. Glucose is catabolized down even further to facilitate the needed phosphate group. Besides glucose, fatty acids can be further broken down for this purpose and, if absolutely necessary, proteins can also be catabolized for this function. Proteins are not the preferred source for the body to utilize, however. First glucose will be catabolized to provide anabolism the necessary building blocks, then fatty acids, and proteins only as a last resort.

Understanding the actual process your body uses to provide for its energy needs tells you something about how you should eat. Diets that eliminate carbs are eliminating the primary source of energy your body is designed to utilize. Certainly we should not overbalance our carb intake, but eating adequate, and properly selected, carbs is absolutely essential for your highest level of health and vitality.

Fact #3 - Your Body Throws Away What It Does Not Need

This fact is critically important for you to understand. You eat food. Your body breaks that food down into its most basic components, and uses those components to create whatever it needs to survive and thrive. Your body breaks some of those components down even further to provide energy via the ATP/ADP cycle. Whatever is left over is thrown away as waste.

And right here you may again be throwing up your hands and objecting. If your body throws away superfluous Legos, that is to say any extra building blocks, remaining after catabolization and anabolization are complete as waste, why do we get fat? Isn't fat stored energy? Doesn't the body save everything and, if we eat more than we use, pack it away as body fat for later use?

No, it does not. At least, not in the way you think it does.

There is perhaps more misinformation bloating blogs and media releases about this one point than any other, and all the misinformation is leading the public to make very poor food choices. If you provide your body with what it requires and eliminate poisonous substances from your diet, your body will use what it needs and quite literally eliminate the excess as waste.

Cellular biologists learn more about this phenomenon every day. Take cholesterol as an example. Only about 25 percent of the cholesterol used by your body comes from food sources. The remaining 75 percent is synthesized by your liver. If the liver makes too much, the excess is eliminated as waste. Cholesterol unused by your body's cells is also returned to the liver, where it is converted to bile salts and eliminated in the feces. If there is an elevated level of cholesterol in the blood, then it is because cholesterol is required to fulfill its primary functions of healing injury or building cells. Excess is always eliminated unless there is a reason for its continued existence. When elevated cholesterol is present, it is more important to discern why the body needs it and address that cause. Taking drugs to reduce cholesterol without addressing the cause of that increased need may very well cause more harm than it cures.

Excess body fat is also eliminated as waste. There is no necessity for it to be burned, and in fact it never is. Excess fat is simply thrown away by the body. If it is instead being stored, it is because your body has an imbalance, a state of malnutrition that your body perceives as a crisis.

To better understand this third fact about how food is used in your body, let's take a closer look at the two types of fat, how they work, and why they exist.

Chapter Eight
A Tale of Two Fats

Did you know there are two types of fat in your body?

Subcutaneous fat is soft and jiggly and resides just under your skin. It also tends to mingle in with muscle tissue. This is the fat you see when you look in the mirror. Despite the fact that most people do not like looking at it, and despite the fact that this is the fat many people fight so hard to lose, it is not especially dangerous. It causes very few serious health problems unless the mass is heavy enough to over-stress your joints and your skeletal structure.

Visceral fat, by contrast, is very dense, nearly solid. It is found inside your abdominal cavity surrounding your vital organs. A certain amount of visceral fat is necessary for health and vitality. However, too much of this fat can be responsible for diabetes, hypertension, heart disease, fatty liver disease, colon cancer, kidney failure, and more.

Misunderstanding these two very different types of fat has led to poor health decisions and all sorts of suffering. Our vanity often gets the best of us as human beings, causing us to make decisions to *look better* before we consider what will make us *feel better* or, more importantly, *be better*. I personally like to believe that if only people **knew better** they would make better decisions. It is with this hope and prayer that I write this chapter.

You hear a lot in the media about "belly fat." In terms of marketing, this phrase is a goldmine. Everyone is talking about exercises, supplements, diets, and surgeries supposedly targeted toward belly fat. In the image on page 57, though, you can see that it is not that simple. The fat outside of your abdominal muscles (abs) is subcutaneous. The fat inside, around, and near your internal organs is visceral fat, the dangerous kind.

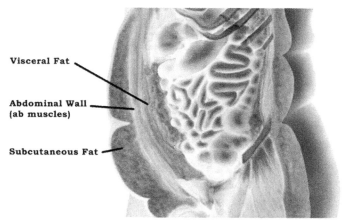

Visceral Fat

Abdominal Wall
(ab muscles)

Subcutaneous Fat

THE DIFFERENCE BETWEEN *VISCERAL* AND *SUBCUTANEOUS* FAT

I believe the path to easier, sustainable, healthy, and honest weight loss is to eat properly. Period. This image will help you understand exactly what I mean, and why I so passionately convey this point of view. We will refer back to this picture throughout the chapter. Let's take a peek at popular weight loss methods, and learn why they fail you in terms of health and wellness.

Weight Loss Surgical Procedures

New weight loss procedures emerge constantly. Liposuction has been around for many years and remains a Hollywood favorite, but is by no means the only fat-removing procedure out there. The ranks have been joined more recently by low-level laser procedures and *cool sculpting*, which freezes fat cells.

All procedures which target specific areas of fat, belly fat in particular, suffer the exact same limitation: they can only address subcutaneous fat. In other words, they may have some level of short term success in making you *look* thinner in the mirror, but they do not and cannot address visceral fat, which is the stuff that is making America sicker and sicker.

The most dangerous aspect of weight loss procedures targeting subcutaneous fat is this: because a person looks better in the mirror, they can easily think they *are* better, and take no further steps toward their overall wellness. Tragically and irresponsibly, doctors and practitioners selling these services market themselves as "wellness" clinics, further deceiving a desperate public.

What about procedures that are more invasive, bariatric surgeries such as stomach staples, gastric bypass, and gastric banding? Such procedures directly affect the delivery of food to the body and therefore can address both visceral and subcutaneous fat, right?

Caveat Emptor. Buyer beware.

If, in fact, the metabolism burned off calories as we are constantly told, these invasive surgeries should work. But they don't work in the long term, and they very often cause even more damage and suffering to recipients.

One of the most common of these surgeries is laparoscopic adjustable gastric banding, a procedure in which a silicone sleeve filled with saline solution is fitted around a portion of the stomach and inflated in order to restrict the passage of food. According to the National Institutes of Health (NIH), "Although early reports described a 35 percent initial excess weight loss on average by most patients, more recent reports describe not only high failure rates but also high reintervention rates for both band-related complications (e.g. band erosion, leakage, slippage, port infection and esophageal dilatation) and failure to lose weight."[20]

That is the least invasive of the surgical procedures and considered among the safest. As procedures become more invasive, they also carry higher risk, up to and including death from the surgery. Many patients suffer severe vomiting, inability to eat nutrient dense foods like green vegetables, abdominal upset, and worse.

Surgical procedures all promise to be the panacea of weight loss success and easy long-term maintenance. I have heard doctors on every major network news and talk show assert that surgery is the only viable option for people with more than 100 pounds to lose. They all cite research studies to support their claims, but those studies are often conducted and paid for by the surgical industry itself.[21] Once third party studies are conducted, such as the NIH report above, actual results prove to be abysmal.

Look, I am going to give you the number one reason to avoid weight loss surgeries right here and right now. Buried deep in the FAQ on all bariatric surgery websites is *The Diet*: the eating plan you are supposed to follow post-operation if you hope to succeed long-term. Doctors who perform weight loss surgeries seldom talk openly about the post-op eating plan. They provide it to patients along with a thick stack of other paperwork that probably never gets read. After your initial weeks of drinking a liquid diet of ultra-processed, chemical-laden stuff, you are instructed to begin eating lean proteins and nutrient-dense vegetables and fruits, and to avoid sugary drinks and processed toxic foods. You are instructed to speak with both psychiatrists and nutritionists to learn mindful eating, to stop eating when full, and to achieve a balance of food types.

And therein lies the rub. After spending $10,000 and more, it is an *eating plan* that ultimately facilitates weight loss and long-term weight management. The two primary reasons weight loss surgeries fail is because patients either did not understand the diet element before getting the surgery, or because they find they cannot follow it afterward.

The inexcusable wholesale tendency of weight loss surgeons to promote surgery while downplaying necessary dietary changes costs patients tens of thousands of dollars apiece; creates weeks, months, or sometimes years of serious eating complications; and causes an exceedingly high rate of weight recurrence. The average weight lost after surgery is seldom more than 55 percent of the excess weight a patient started with, and nearly 80 percent will regain at least some of that.[22]

Contrast that with Tony, who decided to delay his doctor's advice of surgery and consulted with Nutri-90 first. Tony weighed 424 pounds when I began working with him as his wellness coach. By creating a balanced eating plan alone, Tony lost 231 pounds in just over 15 months! Today, three years later, he still weighs 194 pounds. Imagine that: Tony lost 100 percent of his excess weight and hasn't gained any back by following a proper eating plan alone. Isn't that what wellness ought to look like?

Exercise Programs and Gyms

Referring back to the diagram on page 57, it is important to discuss so-called "spot exercises" and their alleged effect on belly fat. Please understand that there is no such thing as targeted fat loss. In other words, an exercise cannot cause belly fat to be lost before other fat, nor to be lost faster than fat from other areas. This is such common knowledge that it doesn't even require a citation. It has never been true and never will be true, and has only ever been a marketer's ploy to separate desperate people from their money.

Right this moment, a thousand voices are being raised in unison to wage battle upon my assertion. So here's the thing: exercises *can* target muscle groups, and exercises that target the abdominal muscles may reduce a person's girth, making it *appear* that they have lost belly fat. But have they?

There are two possibilities. It is becoming more and more accepted that my assertion from a decade ago is, in fact, true: weight loss does not come from exercise; it comes from proper eating. Remember, calories are not a thing in your body and therefore exercise cannot burn them. Weight loss comes from eating the proper balance of foods for your body. So if a person begins an exercise program targeting abdominal muscles and also begins a corrected eating plan, one possibility is that they may well be losing weight all over their body, including, proportionately, their belly.

However, the other possibility is more likely in the case of a gym-goer who has not also improved their eating plan, and it is insidiously dangerous. By strengthening abdominal muscles—especially if done in a program of "core training" that also strengthens all the muscle groups of the core—that visceral fat, the dangerous one, is held back like waters behind a dam. A person's waist can become dramatically smaller because the muscles of the abdominal wall have become stronger, while their abdomen still contains the same volume of a very dangerous substance.

I am certainly not opposed to core training. Quite the opposite; I advocate for it, provided that it is paired with an eating plan appropriate to you which will eliminate excess visceral fat. Beware the trainers who try to sell you on spot-reducing belly fat; they are not trainers to be trusted.

Weight Loss Drugs & Supplements

There exists a glut of drugs and supplements alleged to assist weight loss efforts. Every new pill, powder, or potion to come along alleges it has a "solid scientific basis" along with a whole lot of "research" to back it up. Most often, though, the research is bought and paid for by the company or industry it represents and is grossly misrepresentative, and the science is bogus. Each one grabs attention, sells a great many units, and builds a following, but then it doesn't work, at best, or maybe even gets itself banned for false advertising claims. In some cases, the supplement itself is found to be dangerous to the user.

Don't be fooled by weight loss supplements. The very best reasoning I can offer you to remain un-duped by slick marketing tactics is this, and whether you believe life got here by evolution or by creation, you must arrive at this same conclusion: pills, powders, and potions did not evolve and neither did God create them. Real, honest food, the kind that comes from farms and not factories, is for your body. Pills, powders, and potions are for corporate profit. There is no exception. Ever.

Supplements are, one by one, proven ineffective over time. Each one says they are different. However, in time they are proven to be exactly the same.

But what about FDA-approved weight loss drugs?

Remember your Legos? Legos can be joined to Legos, but not to sticks, stones, and other unrecognizable pieces of broken stuff. When you put chemicals into your body, either via your food, drink, or drugs, you create an internal crisis wherein the chemicals prevent your body from doing something. Most weight loss drugs are suppressing something intentionally: appetite, absorption of food, digestive processes, or even the absorption of fats in the colon. Whenever a natural body function is suppressed there are side effects, and they are neither pleasant nor healthy.

For instance, suppressing the absorption of fats by extension suppresses the absorption of fat-soluble nutrients like Vitamin D that are essential to proper body function. Suppressing appetite by extension suppresses the ingestion of *all* nutrients, and is usually compounded by building cravings for the wrong foods when you do become hungry.

Other side effects can include everything from diarrhea to headaches to intestinal cramps... all the way up to kidney failure and death in extreme cases. When weight loss can be accomplished relatively easily with just the proper use of food, why risk those awful side effects?

One last word on weight loss drugs and surgeries: all of the interventions aimed at restricting the amount of food a person can eat or preventing absorption are designed to prevent calories from getting into your body. I want you to remember right here that no one ever got fat from calories. You know that now. So if those drugs and operations are not restricting calories, what are they restricting?

I have a number of clients in my Nutri-90 wellness program who have endured failed weight loss surgeries. Getting well is very difficult for them, more so than for anyone else. Why? Because surgeries restrict the passage and absorption of *food*, even nutritious food. When a post-op patient tries to adopt a balanced eating plan consisting of real, whole foods from the earth, they find they cannot eat much of it because of the surgical procedure. They can no longer put the proper Legos into their body. How tragic to have been sold a bill of goods by a money-hungry weight loss surgeon, only to find that eating the way we are biologically designed to eat is no longer an option for you. If this is your situation, I can and will help you, but know that yours will be a harder path. Your struggle touches my heart.

Belly Fat vs. Belly Fat

From this point forward, when you hear someone in the media, a blog writer, a so-called expert, or even your doctor talk about "belly fat," I want you to *hear* "visceral fat." It is so easy these days to address and eliminate subcutaneous fat from your belly by sitting in a chair in some clinic under a low-energy laser or *freeze gun*. But when you hear about the dangers of belly fat, subcutaneous fat is not what they are talking about. They are talking about visceral fat, and there is no effective way to eliminate the excess except by proper eating. No other healthy method exists.

Have you ever been to a gym and seen someone using body calipers to determine their body fat percentage? Have you ever seen a bio-feedback scale that has a percent body fat readout? Or have you ever seen the "pinch an inch" commercial, advocating for weight loss if you can pinch more than an inch of body fat on your waist? All of these things measure subcutaneous fat in one form or another. They all measure the thing that is not especially dangerous. Despite the inherent shortcomings of the BMI, or Body Mass Index, it remains one of the easiest means for a regular person to affordably get an idea of their optimal body weight while taking into account both types of fats: subcutaneous and visceral.

Remember, no matter how much you may dislike seeing it in the mirror, subcutaneous belly fat is not really hurting you.

Visceral belly fat, by contrast, may be killing you if you have too much of it.

I keep saying "too much of it" or "excess" when talking about visceral fat. Why? The thing is, some visceral fat is essential to your health and well-being, your overall wellness. Visceral fat provides cushioning for your internal organs, keeping them all in place and isolated from the bumps and jars your body may endure. Visceral fat is also the primary means of storing digested carbs for later use.

Yes, I did say that. While calories are not a thing in the body, the ATP/ADP cycle, or cellular respiration, does require glucose to recharge. Your body will store a certain amount of material that can be easily converted to glucose within your visceral fat deposits. Remember, though, that so long as you are providing your body with the Legos it requires and keeping it free of sticks, stones, and unrecognizable pieces of broken stuff—that is to say, free of processed poisons that do not belong in your body anyway—then your metabolism will throw away what it does not need, and that includes *excess* subcutaneous and visceral fat.

It is not your goal, then, to remove all body fat, nor even "as much as you can." It ought to be your goal to achieve the optimum body configuration for *you*. We will learn later that your body will self-regulate to keep you at your optimal body weight if we only give it a fighting chance.

Chapter Nine
The Way Things Are
(Section Summary)

You are learning a lot about the first step of common sense, "seeing things the way they [really] are." Let's review a bit, okay?

1- Your metabolism does not "burn" anything. Catabolism takes your food apart into its smallest usable pieces and anabolism reassembles them into whatever your body requires. Like Legos, your metabolism builds, repairs, and nourishes every type of cell in your body with the building blocks provided by your food. If your food does not provide all of the necessary building blocks, then your cells will not be structured in the finest fashion for your well-being.

2- Because your metabolism does not burn anything, calories are not a thing in your body. Calories are a unit of measure, not a physical object, and as such, they measure the heat produced by incinerating a substance. Without heat released from incineration there is nothing for a calorie to measure. By virtue of not being physical objects, calories cannot be eaten, stored, burned, or used in any other way.

3- Your body's energy needs come from a process called cellular respiration which utilizes a high energy molecule known as ATP, the energy currency of the body. This process occurs in every cell in your body and uses only a very small portion of the food you eat.

4- There are two types of fat in your body: visceral and subcutaneous. Subcutaneous fat is the stuff you may not like to see in the mirror, but the visceral fat inside your abdominal cavity is the more dangerous stuff. It can only be effectively eliminated by eating the proper balance of real, honest foods and avoiding ultra-processed foods filled with toxic chemicals and devoid of nature-made nutrients.

5- Weight loss surgeries, supplements, drugs, and "targeted exercises" all fail to provide long-term effective weight loss.

There is one more aspect to the way things really are, and it is important to understand it before you can easily see how things ought to be done and fulfill the terms of common sense. We will explore this most treacherous aspect in the next section.

SECTION III

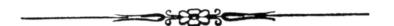

"Economic history is a never-ending series of episodes based on falsehoods and lies, not truths. It represents the path to big money. The object is to recognize the trend whose premise is false, ride that trend, and step off before it is discredited."

George Soros

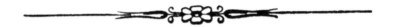

Chapter Ten
The Information Chain

When you read the quote at the beginning of this Section, does it disturb you? Do you find it difficult to believe that much of our economy is based on lies?

Every time I take a marketing class it makes me ill. Truly ill; sick to my stomach. Marketing classes teach manipulation of the highest order, as in, "how can companies more completely manipulate consumers to the degree that the consumer will pay money for whatever companies have to sell, even if it harms them?"

The idea that a person or business would make lots of money selling a lie should not be surprising to anyone by now. The tobacco industry sold death in a stick for more than a hundred years while soliciting professional spokespeople of all stripes, including scientists, doctors, and other medical professionals, to get in front of the public and proclaim cigarettes safe. Marlboro, among others, was considered a "trusted brand." More recently, the mortgage industry drove the U.S. economy nearly to the brink of total destruction by selling home loans that could not possibly be repaid, all the while telling consumers they were a safe path to a bigger, better house for the same money. Those lenders received the interest—their profit margins—first. Then they were there to foreclose upon the loan when it predictably went into default. And finally, they were there to demand and receive the largest government bailout check of all time. They got their profit, they got your collateral, and they got money from the government. And most of those institutions are still operating, still considered to be "trusted brands."

The advice George Soros proffered is considered by many to be the best business advice ever given because it works. If a businessperson identifies a lie that is so simple and reasonable that it can be made believable, and then sells that lie with the support of scientists, doctors, and other professionals, the lie can make a lot of money. A whole lot of money.

The trick has always been to obtain the support of people in whom the public places their trust. In the case of Big Food companies, doctors and scientists are the best representatives, because every American child has been taught from birth to trust men and women in science and medicine.

Therefore, we see doctors who have never taken a single course in nutrition on TV telling us about all of the wonderful "health benefits" of some new supplement, pill, or allegedly heart-conscious food item. We have doctors on TV sporting their most trustworthy white lab coats or scrubs while pushing every sort of supplement and pill, but never advocating for real, honest, farm-fresh foods.

In 2015, TV talk show host Dr. Mehmet Oz appeared on the US Senate floor, admitting that the weight loss products he pushes on his show "don't have the scientific muster" to pass as fact.[23] Sound familiar? Those words mimic what George Soros was saying, don't they? Americans, and indeed much of the developing world, are desperate for weight loss and for improved health. There is little money to be made in the truth, but there are billions of dollars to be made selling weight loss lies, and greedy businesspeople are going to ride that wave until it is discredited. And when it is discredited it won't even matter to business, since their money will have already been made. Only you will pay the price, and right now Americans are paying that price to the tune of more than $60 billion per year!

Part of seeing things as they really are involves understanding why the world is still talking about calories when they so clearly are not a thing in your body. The answer is business and marketing. Money.

The vast majority of the average American's nutritional knowledge has not been delivered by science, but rather by marketing. In 2009, the FDA delivered a warning letter to General Mills because the labeling of Cheerios proclaimed it was a clinically proven, bona fide treatment for high cholesterol.[24] Eventually General Mills changed its labeling, but only as much as necessary to skirt the law. Its labeling to this day promotes Cheerios as a heart healthy product. Because most Americans see General Mills as a trusted brand, consumers take such labeling at face value, believing Cheerios is a truly healthy product to put on the family table.

The number one job of a high-value marketing firm is to create brand trust and brand loyalty. Marketers know that once a brand is perceived as honest and trustworthy, they can sell almost anything just by placing key words on the product's front label. Words like heart healthy, low cholesterol, low fat, organic, natural, anti-oxidant, gluten-free, and the like have been proven to boost consumer product sales over and over again, even when they appear on clearly unhealthy foods.

There is no more profitable term to put on a food product than "low-cal" or "low-calorie." Marketers keep the term alive because it makes a seemingly solid argument in favor of the most treacherous lie in the entire food industry. That lie is this: "All foods are okay if eaten in moderation." By putting calories to the fore, food marketers argue that even the most egregious foods are okay in moderation so long as you as a consumer keep your total calorie consumption down to 2,000 calories per day and exercise to keep your calories in balance.

But calories are not a thing. The worst of the worst foods are killing people not because of some mystical "energy balance," but because they have none of the Legos your body needs to use as building blocks and are instead packed to the gills with poisonous chemicals: sticks, stones, and unrecognizable pieces of broken stuff.

The funny thing is this: we as consumers, by and large, absolutely know that processed foods are not healthy and that they cause obesity, heart disease, and numerous other debilitating diseases. Collectively, we call these the diseases of civilization. And yet we still fall for slick marketing tactics and deceitful product labeling, driving sales of junk food to ever higher heights. As hard as it is to mentally absorb, Americans eat, on average, 3 fast food burgers every week. That means every man, woman and child in the country.[25]

Some clients come to me and let me know straight away that they eat better than most folks and already have a head start, as it were, to truly healthy eating. That almost always means they buy only foods with healthy-looking front labels. And that also almost always means they are just eating a more expensive processed poisonous chemical.

There is an ancient Latin phrase that applies here: *caveat emptor*. This phrase literally means "let the buyer beware," and is used in law to acknowledge that the seller of a thing generally has more knowledge about it than the buyer, but it is the buyer's responsibility to inform themselves before purchase and they cannot hold the seller liable after sale. While we do have laws that supposedly protect the buyer of consumer food products in America, those laws are based on the 175-year-old archaic belief in calories, and therefore offer little to no real consumer protection.

Doctors, Nutritionists, and Registered Dietitians

I think most people would acknowledge that food companies are not entirely above board about the contents of their products. But what about doctors? Aren't doctors in the know and able to advise patients on nutrition? The sad truth is... no, they aren't. At the time of this writing, only 26 universities turning out doctors in America even offer a dedicated nutrition course, and it is not a required class in many of those. [26] The vast majority of American doctors barely study nutrition; it is not a part of the Medical Doctor (MD) degree. Doctors very often rely, then, on the same published reports that you do, or on nutritionists and Registered Dietitians.

The major problem with the Registered Dietitian (RD) and Registered Dietitian Nutritionist (RDN) certifications in America is the Academy of Nutrition and Dietetics (AND), the national authority for the certifications. The AND accepts money for partnerships with big food corporations and their marketers and lobbyists. These include and have included the likes of the American Beverage Association, National Dairy Council, General Mills, and even straight up purveyors of obesity like McDonalds. The AND argues that such partnerships actually advance the cause of nutrition by bringing the food industry to the table and promoting healthier choices. However, the California branch of the national association, the California Dietetic Association (CDA), served up McDonalds at their own 2014 annual convention in deference to the "gold-level" contribution the Golden Arches made to the association.[27] Why is that a big deal? Because that convention is where California nutritionists and dietitians go to keep up on their continuing education credits. The example set in such a setting matters. At the time of this writing, a splinter of AND members operate a group called Dietitians for Professional Integrity, which is dedicated to breaking the influential connections between the food industry and the AND.[28]

When a food company gives sponsorship money to an organization like the AND, especially if it's a large amount, that money buys something. In this case, it buys a foot in the door to provide "educational materials" to our nation's nutritionists and dietitians and to contribute to the course materials used in educating new pupils to the certification. It is no accident that nutritionists, like Big Food marketers, universally fall back on calories, promoting the notion that anything is okay to eat in moderation so long as calories are kept in balance.

Surely scientists can be trusted, though, right? Unfortunately, no. *Vice News* recently completed a four-part series entitled "Science for Sale" documenting the powerful influence of industry in contemporary scientific research, in which findings favor industry 96 out of 100 times.[29] While Vice's feature did not address food science directly, money is a very powerful tool and science in all fields has largely succumbed. Far too often, even studies that have been peer-reviewed are not trustworthy.

As a result of the tainting of these entire professions, scientists, nutritionists, dietitians, and doctors fall back on calories, and they prescribe medications, programs, devices, surgeries, and drugs that all purport to reduce excess calories in the body. Is it any wonder that the industrialized world is getting fatter and fatter? No, they are not getting fat from calories; they are getting fat because their bodies are malnourished; they do not have the building blocks to keep them heathy and fit, nor do they have the knowledge to correct that deficiency.

Chapter Eleven
The Ugly Underbelly of Marketers

In the marketing courses I have taken personally, I have learned one thing above all else: the products lining the shelves of your nearest supermarket are there because you put them there. Market research is a process that rapes the minds and souls of the population, strips off the veils of propriety, removes the masks through which we see ourselves, and lays bare the naked biological processes that drive us. The items that line the shelves are there because we, collectively, cannot resist them. They are us, the populace, laid bare and naked.

Food makers know the substances that cause addiction. They know the cravings those addictions create physiologically. They know how to manufacture those substances cheaply and efficiently and how to disguise them in products you would never suspect. Marketers know how to create needs in people, needs that once never existed but which now cannot be denied.

These two forces—addiction and perceived need leading to feelings of deprivation—when combined form a powerful enemy to be reckoned with. Yet even though they are the enemy, people hand over their money quite willingly.

Do you think I am exaggerating? Ask the client who bought Hostess donuts, which she would eat by the boxful. Feeling guilty for devouring the very thing she knew was the downfall of her health and wellness, she threw them out. Then, against every will of her mind, she pulled them out of the trash and ate them. All of them. This was her experience three or more times every week.

You might think this example is extreme, but do a little people watching next time you are at the supermarket. How many already-obese people are entering the checkout line with cases of soda alongside bagged and boxed junk food laden with flour, sugar, and fats of dubious origin? How many have carts full of prepared meals rather than fresh fruits, vegetables, and meats? Many, if not most, of those people know intellectually that their food choices are robbing them of their health, but they don't know how to reclaim control of their life from their food. They can't resist buying the very stuff that is destroying the quality of their lives. It is little different than the driving dynamic of a drug addict or alcoholic, except in the case of toxic foods there is no help from the powers that be.

Here is a surprising fact: the process used by food marketers to create such widespread addiction and destructive behavior is remarkably simple and relatively easy to set up. Psychologists call it *classical conditioning*. To better understand classical conditioning, though, let's briefly explore a specific kind of addiction: cravings.

Cravings

Cravings can be wickedly powerful. I have clients who become outright angry and almost verbally abusive when fighting through cravings. There are even words and phrases being coined for this, words like "hangry." This word is less about 'hungry and angry' than it is about the incredible power of cravings.

Cravings these days are accepted as a natural part of the human condition—something everyone experiences, something normal. But are they really normal? The answer is no. There are certain rare cravings that result from specific bodily needs, but if you think about the symptoms of your cravings and how they affect you both psychologically and physically, you can quickly spot two parallels that ought to cause you to step back and think carefully. Most cravings are really *addiction* and *conditioning* in disguise.

Addiction and conditioning are not normal. Addiction is brought on by putting offending substances in your body, while conditioning, in the context of food, is a form of brainwashing very purposefully planned and executed by someone against you, often for the purpose of greater profit for themselves. Let's make a quick examination of each of these phenomena with an eye toward the way you eat and those painful cravings that so often kill weight loss efforts.

Addiction

Addiction comes in two forms:
1. substances which are physically addictive, and
2. psychological addiction, which often stems from strong emotional events, memories, or connections.

Physical addiction is the most prevalent food addiction, and is the result of either (or both!) additives in our foods or hyper-concentration of certain food components through processing. Although we speak jokingly about being "addicted" to our favorite foods, it is no joke; addictive food elements trigger the same chemical responses in the brain as heroin, morphine, and cocaine![30]

Sometimes the addictive substance appears on the ingredient label and sometimes not. MSG (monosodium glutamate) is used extensively in foods as a flavor enhancer, and it is highly addictive. It appears as an ingredient on food labels, as do many other chemical additives that are known to be addictive, although they often appear with cleverly confusing names. But why are we so easily addicted to other "whole foods" whose ingredient labels show only wholesome ingredients? That is because of processing. While there are hundreds of examples, let's consider just two.

Casein. Casein is a protein naturally found in milk, and is not normally addictive in its natural state. Strip it out of milk and concentrate it, though, and it becomes extremely addictive. Do you crave cheese? Many people do, yet the ingredient label usually shows only healthful ingredients. Remembering that cravings are, in fact, addictive responses makes us dig deeper to understand why our cravings can be so strong. In this case, refined, concentrated casein is the reason. It can be added to cheeses in its refined, addictive state and still be called simply "milk" on the ingredient list because it is the primary protein of milk. Tricky, right? Most commercial cheese makers are just that tricky, though, because making you addicted makes them money. The same trickery is used to add casein to French fries which contain other milk-derived ingredients, burger buns, milk shakes, baked goods, other types of desserts, creamy salad dressings, whipped toppings, sausages, and more. We will talk more about casein in later chapters.

Gluten. Like casein, gluten is a protein, this time one found primarily in wheat. Modern flour is processed in such a way as to strip down and hyper-concentrate gluten, making this protein an addictive substance. Once food scientists discovered this secret addictive property of concentrated gluten, it was incorporated into the processing of flour and put into as many foods as possible, from breakfast sausage to certain hot sauces and even ice cream. Flour is the primary ingredient in some fast food French fries and potato chips, as well as in everything breaded, which seems to be almost everything in Americanized "Chinese" foods, fast foods, and deli offerings.

It doesn't stop there, though, not by a long shot. There are literally scores of addictive substances added to the processed food supply. There is a reason "no one can eat just one," and obesity is the tangible result of a population addicted to the food additives infesting nearly every food product encountered, both in-home and out.

The remedy for physical addiction is to eliminate processed, packaged foods as much as possible. This isn't necessarily easy; in the process you may encounter addictive responses similar to those of a drug addict, including very strong cravings, but you can do it and getting clean will be one of the best decisions you ever make.

Psychological food addiction is a mixed bag of physiological addiction and psychological food relationships and connections. Sometimes the help of a professional psychotherapist is required in treating psychological food addiction, but not always, and there are plenty of positive actions you can implement on your own.

The first is to realize that many words commonly used with regards to weight loss, words like "cheat" and "faithful," are destructive words linked to sin, shame, and guilt. These are the same words we use when talking about spousal relationships and religion. But food is a thing, not a relationship. Consciously stop using those words and instead realize that food is a decision, and as such has a consequence we will either like or not, depending on the decision we make.

Other strategies for psychological food addiction include:
- Be fully present in each moment. Perhaps even try meditating to remove past and future feelings of guilt or worry.

- Accept your current life situation; you can work toward future successes while still accepting and finding thankfulness for where you currently are in life.
- Be active in new and interesting ways, changing the scenery and being very careful to avoid food in the new activities in order to stay clear of new food associations.
- Relax. Find a place you do not usually sit or lie down, and use that spot for relaxation and meditation, keeping it free of any food or drink except water or tea.
- Be curious and resolve to explore and contemplate life's mysteries.

Conditioning or "Classical Conditioning"

Classical conditioning is an entire field of psychological study, and precious little of it works to your benefit. I am only going to share one small part of it here, but it will be enough for you to appreciate how deeply we have been manipulated and even outright brainwashed to eat more and more.

More than a hundred years ago, at the turn of the twentieth century, a man named Ivan Pavlov was doing work that would eventually change the course of food marketing forever. Pavlov's work later became known as *classical conditioning*. You may have heard of *Pavlov's dogs*, which were the subject of his experiments, somewhere along your life's journey.

In short, here is what Pavlov did and what he learned. Pavlov measured the excretions of saliva and gastrointestinal fluids when dogs ate. Most interesting in his later findings were the excretions *before* the animals ate, because these were associated with the drive to find and eat food. Finding food is a primal and very powerful drive in all living things.

In his experiments, Pavlov would play a metronome or ring a bell whenever the dogs were fed. The dogs made an association between the sounds and the acquisition of food. After some time, Pavlov made the sounds but did not bring food. The dogs began to excrete saliva and digestive fluids simply at the sound, even without the presence of food.

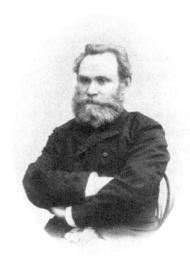

IVAN PAVLOV
Reprinted from
U.S. National Library of Medicine

Then Pavlov went one step further: he would make the sounds 30 minutes *after* the dogs had eaten, a time when they clearly would not be hungry in any biological sense. Even when not hungry, the dogs began to excrete fluids and actively look for food after hearing the sounds. When food could not be found, the dogs would become aggressive to their handlers, and would not back down until food was provided!

Finally, something happened that was not part of the experiment, and that something was very telling in terms of how we work psychologically. Pavlov discontinued the experiments after having documented his findings. What he hadn't realized was that the dogs were no longer listening only to the bells and metronomes; they had actually begun registering his footsteps and seeking food as soon as they heard him coming. That singular connection, that conditioning between Pavlov's footsteps and food, was so powerful as to affect the moods and behavior of the dogs in negative and destructive ways. Remember "hangry"?

It should be no surprising secret what food makers and marketers have learned from Pavlov's experiments. People, like Pavlov's dogs, could be *conditioned* to look for food, even when they are not hungry in any physical sense! As early as the 1970s, but very aggressively beginning in the 1980s, major food companies began a different type of marketing, one that took a very long-term view of market share. They began marketing to kids with an eye toward gaining their loyalty as adults. They did this successfully, and are still doing so today, using classical conditioning techniques: creating powerful associations between events, places, emotions, and food while people are still young, conditioning that will carry strongly into adulthood.

And so it is today that people look for food almost always and everywhere, even when they are clearly not hungry in the primal sense. Folks will eat dinner and then, less than an hour later, order a gallon of popcorn and a quart or more of soda at the movies. They might even go out for ice cream after that. We will eat at events no matter how full we are just because we are offered cake by a host or hostess. We will eat in the car, at the mall, at the beach, while walking, and on and on. And not only that, we will seek the largest portion of food or drink that is available. It is mindless eating, meaning we do not think about it, and we often aren't even aware of it. Have you ever tried to write a list of every morsel you ate the previous day? It can be really difficult because so much of our eating is mindless; we do it without thought.

Classical conditioning is blatant manipulation, even brainwashing. Preventing its influence over you starts by becoming aware of what it is, consciously learning to recognize it in advertising and marketing, and then allowing yourself to become angry that you have been so manipulated. When angry, it becomes much easier to consciously take a stand against it. Consciously eat at meal times, and consciously avoid eating when the only reason for it is where you are, who you are with, or what is happening around you.

Think, for a moment, of your own strong cravings. Are they the result of addiction or of conditioning? In many cases, your strong cravings are the result of both. Start by recognizing and accepting what cravings really are. Do you remember how, earlier in this book, I stressed that words mean things? If you call your impulses toward food "cravings," you mentally write them off as natural, normal, and something to be flirted with via "cheat days," or by feeling that you "deserve" it. If, on the other hand, you call them by their real and true name, *addictions*, you are more likely to avoid them, knowing that even a little bit can easily lead to binging and other unhealthy habits.

Knowledge is power, and knowing this about addictions gives you a place and a means to start the process of getting your body clean.

Marketers and Calories

Marketers have three main tasks. The first is to get you to believe a need exists where none may have existed before, even making you feel deprived if you do not have whatever thing they are selling. A hundred years ago, by way of example, there was no such thing as a TV. Today it is considered a necessity, by law in most states. In some areas, a household is considered to be in a state of poverty if it does not have at least one TV.

In the world of food, just think for a moment: what is the product you "can't live without"? How about coffee creamer? Creamer is a product that generally does not contain an ounce of actual cream; instead, it is chock full of chemical sweeteners, flavors, and preservatives. It is a product that did not exist 50 years ago, but many people use it daily now. They cannot envision a morning without it. Marketers created that "need."

The second job of a marketer is to fill that artificially created need with a product that you will buy not once or twice, but repeatedly, habitually. This is where addiction and classical conditioning come in. In our coffee creamer example, creamers are made, in part, of ingredients engineered to be addictive, and are constantly being updated with new flavors perceived to be exciting or fresh. Tactics like these ensure consumers are never without creamer in their homes. It has become a staple for many.

The third job is to proactively deflect any objection to the product that might arise. This is where marketers enlist the aid of bought-and-paid-for doctors, nutritionists, scientists, or whoever, if needed, to stand up publicly and testify on behalf of a given product, and to belittle anyone who might object. Quite literally in the world of food, these paid "experts" will accuse legitimate science of disingenuous fearmongering while holding up the poisonous product they represent as completely harmless in moderation. A great example is how today's organic produce growers have to legally defend and prove their product, while factory food producers simply make and sell their chemical laden garbage. In the case of our creamer, highly paid lobbyists and "experts" for the food industry and its marketers downplay the detrimental effects of its very unhealthy ingredients, like high fructose corn syrup and hydrogenated oils, with Congress and the various regulatory agencies. They belittle sound science as "scare tactics" and assert no ingredient is "bad" if consumed in moderation.

This third task is also why food marketers and food company lobbyists work diligently, both in legal arenas and in the public eye, to keep calories alive and well in your paradigms—that is to say, your deep belief systems. Calories, you see, are the excuse you use to poison yourself. By believing in calories as the primary value indicator of food, anything and everything becomes okay to eat so long as you "work it off," or eat little enough of it that you do not exceed your daily caloric allotment. If you don't exercise, you may instead move to low-calorie alternatives of your favorite processed foods. So long as you believe in calories, food makers and marketers can and will use that belief against you, slowly killing you for their own profit.

Do you remember the summer of 2014, when Coke built a giant stationary bike people could ride in order to "buy" a coke by first burning the calories to "pay" for it? It was called the *Happy Cycle*, and here is what Coke had to say about it:

> *"What if there were a new, fun way to pay for a Coke? And what if you could do it with your energy? That's exactly what happened when Coca-Cola launched the Happy Cycle and invited people to ride a whimsical bike and trade their calories for a Coke. It's the latest delightful example of Coca-Cola's worldwide stunts that bring people and happiness together."[31]*

This ad would never work without the two key elements we have discussed here: classical conditioning, which Coke has used expertly for decades in order to mentally and emotionally link its soft drinks with happiness; and the ubiquitous belief in calories, which Coke uses to make you believe you can burn off any damage the drink might cause in just a few minutes on a bike.

And that is why counting calories is killing you, America, and much of the world. The damage is not just a couple of extra pounds caused by calories that you can just burn away. The damage caused by highly processed foods and drinks includes diabetes, kidney damage, heart disease, cancer, fatty liver disease, joint degeneration, and more. The damage is caused by the wholesale depletion of nutrients from your food supply and the saturation of that same food supply with chemicals and fillers that do not belong in a human body, not even in some fictional level of moderation. You will not stop and reverse the damage until you stop counting calories and start counting the nutrients, the Legos, which your body needs to survive and thrive.

The longer you believe that calories are a thing in your body, and the longer you believe nutrition, health, and fitness are about caloric "energy balance" and three macro-nutrients, the longer you will be vulnerable to the ridiculous claims of food marketers. And the harder it will be for you to regain your vitality, health, and well-being.

Emotional Eating

In the world of food, emotional eating is closely associated with classical conditioning. Food marketers have not only attached food to virtually every place and event in our collective cultural consciousness, but also to emotions. Americans eat because we are happy, we eat because we are sad, we eat to celebrate, and we eat to mourn. We eat because we are stressed. We eat because we are relieved.

You might think emotional eating is a wholly natural thing that humans have done since the beginning of time. You would be right, but not in the context we think of today.

The term "comfort food" can be traced to a 1966 article in *The Palm Beach Post*. Under the heading "Sad Child May Overeat," it read, "Adults, when under severe emotional stress, turn to what could be called 'comfort food'—food associated with the security of childhood, like mother's poached egg or famous chicken soup."

As long as there have been human beings, there have also been traditions and familial behaviors that accompany life events and the upbringing of children. When children are ill, loving mothers have prepared certain foods, foods that brought comfort—comfort foods. It is normal that adults, when ill, would crave those foods because they are emotionally connected with the love and attention that accompanied them.

That is where the normalcy of modern comfort foods and emotional eating stops, though. Traditionally, mothers made foods for their ill children that had healthy, healing properties, like "mother's poached egg or famous chicken soup." They brought not only mother's comfort, but also nutrition that helped nurse children back to health. Today, people devour pizza, donuts, cookies, pie, and all sorts of nutritionally bankrupt stuff in the name of comfort food. None of this is connected with nurturing mothers and vitality. And curiously, when I ask my clients after a "comfort food binge" if they feel comforted now, the day after, the answer is invariably, "No; I feel much worse, and guilty."

And that is the dangerous differentiation. Comfort food once was food that comforted; you felt better the next day. The junk called comfort food today brings no comfort at all, only shame and grief. How is it that you call it "junk food" in one breath, knowing full well that is exactly what it is, and in the next breath call it "comfort food"?

In this context, marketers have defiled something that once was healthier, and instead created a deadly paradox. Folks are more stressed than ever, and the comfort proffered by marketers to relieve that stress not only leads to unhealthy behaviors, shame, and guilt, but also creates even more stress in its wake. Placing "mother" and "grandma" in product names, evoking images of mom's warmth on product packaging, and producing video advertising featuring warm and happy families sharing food that can only be called absolute junk has gradually eroded mom's love and replaced it with factory-profit-driven, emotion-based classical conditioning.

In the spring of 2012, I received this question from a person interested in the Nutri-90 system:

> "Do any of your successful clients ever cheat during RFL [Nutri-90's Rapid Fat Loss Phase]?"
> ~Serious in Seattle

This was my response:

> It is time I share with you a couple of new ways to think about our relationship with food, okay? First, food is an inanimate object, and therefore not a thing we should be having a relationship with in the first place. Second, you are learning a new way to think about food, your body, and the interaction between the two. It is a philosophical approach; it's also not something you ought to form a relationship with.

Why do I use the word "relationship" here? Because that is the way we talk about food and diet every day. It is deeply ingrained in us, almost from birth, and it adversely affects all of our efforts to be healthy in body, mind, and spirit.

For example, we use words like "faithful" when we stick to a diet plan, and "cheat" when we don't. Those words evoke religion, as though what we eat constitutes righteousness or sin. They are the same words we use when we talk about relationships with a spouse or partner. Does food really belong in the same category?

But seriously, why are those terms bad? Because they evoke shame and guilt if we "cheat," even if we have given ourselves permission to do so. Shame and guilt are entirely negative emotions, serving no useful purpose at all. Shame and guilt lead to feelings of inadequacy, failure, and even depression. Every one of those feelings will kill weight loss dead. How many times have you or someone you know given up on weight loss because of these very feelings?

So here is the thing: there is neither shame nor guilt with Nutri-90. There is neither faithfulness nor cheating. There is neither relationship nor religion. What *is* there, then? There are decisions and consequences, no more and no less. We make decisions, enlightened and empowered by the fact that we are learning the outcome of those decisions before we even make them. Because we know the outcome in advance, we can make a second decision right at the start: the *mitigating decision*, the decision that allows us to deviate from the plan without actually hurting our progress. Does this make sense so far?

Let's take an example: eating out. Is it "cheating" while on a weight loss plan? No, of course it isn't. It is a decision that has a predictable consequence. If you don't mind the consequence, and if you are okay with your progress slowing or even stopping for a few days because of the decision, go for it! Don't feel guilty about the decision. But—and this is important—neither feel ashamed, frustrated, or angry at the predictable consequence when it comes to pass.

You see, the concept of cheating does not allow us to think that way. Cheating, shame, and guilt make us think in absolutes: either we avoid eating out and are "faithful," or we go out and are "cheating." It follows, almost always, that if we choose to cheat, we feel we have already failed, sinned as it were, and therefore we throw all caution to the wind and "just enjoy it"; isn't that true? Or maybe we don't enjoy it at all but instead say, "F**k it, I already messed up; I may as well blow it all the way." But if we let go of the idea that our interaction with food is a religion or a relationship, we free ourselves to make real decisions, decisions that allow us to live and have fun while still successfully accomplishing our goals.

This is just one of the reasons we call Nutri-90 a *wellness plan*, rather than a weight loss or "diet" plan. Your journey should not be about rigidity, rules, and guilt, and it should not be solely about weight loss, either. It should be about gaining a skills set that allows you to manage your weight for the rest of your days, while enjoying this life we live. Even the food. ~BC

Do you discern the import of my response to *Serious in Seattle*? As early as the 1920s, "calories" began to be used as a moral currency, casting judgment against overweight people perceived to be eating too many of them. It soon followed that "diets" were created, ostensibly to help people eat less calories. However, because calories were now irrevocably connected to morality, veering from the diet was unfaithfulness, cheating. Such perceived deviant behavior led to shaming from others along with internal guilt and shame from the cheater themselves.

From then until now, not a single person has ever been able to control their caloric intake well enough. Why? *Because you cannot control that which does not exist.* By keeping the concept of calories, which we now know irrefutably is not a thing in the body at all, in front of the masses as the only element that matters, food marketers have hijacked ultimate moral authority solely for themselves. They are the priests of body mass who will instill guilt and shame for moral caloric deviance and provide absolution if you follow their prescribed penance. Yet the penance is itself based in calories and so cannot be reconciled, and the cycle of shame and guilt spirals ever downward until the majority are overweight or obese, unhappy, stressed, and held captive to a paradigm of food which quite literally condemns them to sickness and death.

Breaking free from this immoral priesthood of marketers is really very simple. Recognize the complex, confusing jumble of nonsense surrounding calories and processed food for what it is: total bunk. Only two things are true:

1. There is no guilt or shame; there are only decisions and the consequences of those decisions, and
2. There are no calories in food whatsoever, only nutrients your body needs, or the absence of those nutrients.

In short, you have a simple decision to make: choose food rich in the 90+ nutrients your metabolism requires to keep you alive and thriving and achieve vitality, fitness, and holistic wellness; or choose nutrient-bankrupt toxic food full of poisonous chemicals and fillers, and achieve chronic illness and utter lack of mobility. The decision becomes exceedingly clear once the cloudy, confusing, manipulative element of calories is removed, doesn't it?

Mechanically, this is very simple. Emotionally, it can be much more complex, but remember that the emotional complexity comes directly from the stress of trying to merge the facts with your pre-existing paradigms, the truth with a misleading fabrication already deeply instilled in your psyche. This phenomenon is called *cognitive dissonance*. Let's talk about it.

Chapter Twelve
Comfortably Numb—The Mind Side

I love the music of Pink Floyd. Pioneers of the concept album, in the 1960s and 1970s they were on the cutting edge of psychological juxtaposition in music. The next time you listen to "Another Brick in the Wall," replace "classroom" with "media" and "teacher" with "marketer." It will open your eyes.

Cognitive Dissonance

Cognitive dissonance is defined as "psychological conflict resulting from simultaneously held incongruous beliefs and attitudes (as a fondness for smoking and a belief that it is harmful)."[32]

Here is a great example of how it works with food:

On one hand, you know soda has no nutritive value at all, contains far too much sugar, and is linked with all sorts of illnesses.

On the other hand, you really love the taste and you want it. In fact, you are driven to have it and can't see not having it. You might say you are addicted to it.

These two thoughts are inconsistent. Not only are they inconsistent, but one of them is a harbinger of doom, and you know it to be true. The human psyche has a built-in control that prohibits a normally adjusted person from committing self-harm, yet you are addicted to this stuff and can't stop drinking it. All of this causes a state of stress in the mind, and that is cognitive dissonance. Somehow, you have to reconcile these two inconsistent thoughts or you will, in a very real sense, begin to go crazy.

Addictive responses are helpful, though, because the addicted brain is open to suggestion. Along come food marketers and their calories to save you.

"Listen," they say, "the danger is in the sugar and calories, right? So just drink diet soda and you will be fine."

Problem solved! Your mind can continue along peacefully.

But then you learn that diet soda contains all sorts of chemicals that kill things in laboratories, and that diet sodas may be worse for diabetes than the regular stuff! Now what?

"No worries," they say. "Have the regular stuff; just work off the calories and you will be fine."

Okay, cool!

This is how your mind works when you are trying to justify the continuance of an unhealthy behavior. Your mind absolutely must connect the points of dissonance, or disagreement, somehow. If you are not addicted to the thing in question, you simply remove one leg of the argument: you stop eating or drinking the thing. However, if you are addicted to the thing, that is not easy to do and you may find yourself open to the suggestions that justify continuing to consume the thing.

Don't fool yourself. You may consciously dupe yourself into believing you can continue the behavior and beat the odds, but subconsciously you know you are playing Russian Roulette: there is a bullet somewhere in the gun you have pointed at your head, and sooner or later it is going to kill you when you pull that trigger. That subconscious knowledge feeds the cycle of guilt, shame, binge "comfort" consumption, resultant guilt, and shame, then more eating and drinking... you get the idea, right? Rotate the chamber, pull the trigger. Repeat.

When my clients reach their weight loss goals, they express many insights to me, things they have learned, experienced, or begun to appreciate, often for the first time in their lives. One universal insight everyone gains is that eating right feels good. It feels good in your body. It feels good in your mind. It feels good emotionally. When you stop eating things that cause a state of cognitive dissonance in your psyche, you start to understand freedom. My clients most often start Nutri-90 believing they want to be free to eat whatever they want; they end their program understanding that they were slaves to food when they started, and eliminating processed junk is the very thing that set their minds free of the stress of cognitive dissonance.

Paradigm Shifts

Remember for a moment the terrifying experience I shared with you at the outset of this book. I awoke on my kitchen floor with my pants soaking wet, staring at the underside of my kitchen cabinets. A few minutes later I was on my way to the emergency room, certain I would not see another sunrise.

That singular experience changed everything for me. Literally everything. The sum of my life from then until now—my research, my work, my writings—are all because of that one event. Nutri-90 (the company I have built to guide others on their journey to wellness), the coaching I have provided to thousands of people just like you, even this book, are all a direct result of that moment of extreme emotional upheaval. Even how I spend vacations and the importance of my family and friends has changed.

By way of reminder, the late Dr. Stephen Covey called this an emotionally based paradigm shift: a singular emotionally charged moment that changes everything about how a person thinks and acts.

I asked myself then, "Why? Why did it take something so dramatic as believing I was dying to get me thinking about my own health and vitality?" In the first chapters of Dr. Covey's book *The 7 Habits of Highly Effective People*, he discusses paradigms and how to change them. You do not have to wake up on the floor to see the world differently. You can *choose* to change your paradigms however you like quite easily. First, though, you need to understand what paradigms are.

I want you to consider this string of facts for a moment:

1. What you believe directs what you think.
2. What you think guides your decision process.
3. What you decide drives what you do, the actions you take.
4. What you do is directly responsible for your outcomes; either they succeed or they do not.

Can you accept each of those statements as true? Good. Because if you connect the dots and condense this down to its simplest form here is what you must also accept:

What you* believe *is directly responsible for your outcomes.

And that explains why some people always seem to get it right while others are perpetually besieged with apparent dead ends and failures: "the rut." While you are struggling so hard to act the right way, to make the correct decisions, or to change your thinking, you are completely missing the piece that drives the entire machine. You must change your paradigms, your deepest beliefs that drive everything you think and do, and hence your outcomes.

Do you wrestle with personal hypocrisies? For example, in the realm of food do you know what you should be eating yet find it really hard to do so? On the flip side, do you understand that what you are putting into your mouth is probably not very good for you, and yet you still keep putting it in there, almost on autopilot? These juxtapositions illustrate a concept you must understand in order to affect change in your life: the subconscious does not think or reason; it simply *does*. Your subconscious is like a computer which can only run programs. Your paradigms are those programs—they subconsciously control your thoughts and actions. The apparent hypocrisy you experience results from the fact that your conscious thoughts are often at odds with your subconscious paradigms, or controlling programs.

In this way, your paradigms are connected with cognitive dissonance. This stressful condition occurs when what you *know* conflicts with what you *believe*. How does this happen? Well, what you know comes from conscious thought and reasoning. It is constantly affected by your changing environment, your information stream, and what you choose to accept as true or reasonable. What you believe, on the other hand, is stored in your subconscious. It does not think nor reason; it simply does. It is a controlling program that runs automatically.

The thing about your paradigms, or those deep, subconscious beliefs that run things on auto-pilot for you, is that you probably did not put them there yourself. They were formed and placed at a very early age by your parents, teachers, church leaders, and peers. Others were placed by highly trained marketers who are extremely adept at manipulating and implanting paradigms. It is their job to do so while keeping you from understanding what they are doing. After all, the less you know about what they are doing, the less likely you are to disbelieve it or to counteract it. The less likely you are to learn how to control yourself and your own outcomes.

So your paradigms are your programming. The subconscious does not reason; it simply does. You have a series of paradigms, or very deep-seated beliefs, that guide a thousand decisions every day that you are not even aware you are making. Some studies estimate people make over 6,000 such decisions every day.[33] This is why you might drive to work, quite safely, and yet have no real memory of how you got there. All of your driving decisions were made on auto-pilot, as it were, completely automatically based on your subconscious programming, or paradigms.

This is also why people eat when they are stressed. More than that, it is why they eat *what* they eat when they are stressed. What to eat and when are programmed paradigms, and you act on them with no conscious thought. People are not crazy when they report there was food going into their mouth and they had no memory of even picking it up, or that certain processed products seemingly appeared in the shopping cart on their own. Your subconscious does it automatically.

So you are screwed, right? Paradigms do not reason; they just do. And how they will respond is programmed almost from birth, so... you are pretty much screwed.

Well… no. While your subconscious does not reason, it can be programmed by your conscious mind—which does reason, or at least *can* reason—if you choose to do so. You can reprogram your paradigms. Here's how:

STEP 1- Make a decision to be aware of a certain aspect of your life. Don't pick everything you want to change all at once; it's too much. Just pick one thing you will be aware of. Write that thing down on paper and tape it to the bathroom mirror, or somewhere else where you will see it every day. When you see it, read and repeat it three times to keep it fresh in your mind.

For example, make a decision to be aware of everything that goes into your mouth. Everything. Write it on paper: "I will be aware and mindful of everything I eat, drink, and suck on today." Tape it to your bathroom mirror and read it every day. Repeat it to yourself three times: "I will be aware and mindful of everything I eat, drink, and suck on today."

STEP 2- Then, as you go through your day, do exactly that; be aware of everything that goes into your mouth. Watch your patterns. Do you eat different things when you are feeling stress or pressure? How are they different? What are you feeling when you reach for foods that sabotage your weight loss or health efforts?

STEP 3- When you become aware that you are putting something in your mouth that you do not want to be there at that particular time, take it back out and consciously tell yourself what you *do* want there. If you are not hungry and don't really want anything there, then tell yourself so. Tell yourself in clear, simple words. When your *inner voice* objects, realize that that inner voice is your programming speaking: your paradigms. That inner voice is the thing you are reprogramming, changing, so never let it win the argument. It cannot reason; it only acts, and so arguing with it is pointless, right? Just tell it what you are going to do and override it.

Curiously, it does not take long to reprogram paradigms if you just follow those three steps. In very short order, you will notice your habits changing as your programming changes. In this example, you will become surprisingly aware of what you consume each day, and powerfully driven to change it. Changing your paradigm means that a thousand little decisions you make every day with no conscious thought will change, too. In just a couple of weeks of concerted effort, you will have changed a paradigm, a habit, for the better, and that change will last for life unless you change it back or allow others, like expert marketers, to do so for you.

The first time I tried this, it honestly pissed me off. After learning these steps, I was assigned this exercise: whenever I saw a piece of trash on the ground and started to walk past it, I was to: 1, notice what I was doing; 2, tell myself "I want to do the right thing just because it is the right thing to do"; and 3, pick up the trash and throw it away.

I did this for about a week very consciously. One day during the second week, I was in a real hurry. I ran past a cup on the ground and BAM: my newly reprogrammed paradigm turned me around to pick up the trash. I consciously told myself I was in a hurry and to forget about it, but the programming was already too strong. It bugged me so much that I walked back about 50 feet to pick the stupid thing up and throw it away. But worse than that, I had told myself I would "do the right thing because it was the right thing to do." That paradigm, worded that way, extended way beyond trash. It was a toppling domino rearranging my entire subconscious and it changed me in so many ways that I cannot even know them all. To this day, I cannot pass a piece of trash on the ground without my conscience pricking me to pick it up and throw it away. And I am constantly telling myself, "do the right thing; it is the right thing to do," when making decisions of all sorts.

Paradigm programming is extremely powerful in human beings. Poorly programmed paradigms make you do a lot of things that are completely wrong for you, because those paradigms have been programmed and implanted by others, not by you. But if you take the time to train yours using these simple steps, they will be equally powerful in leading you to do all the *right* things for you, mostly without you even having to think about them.

Understand this: in one form or another, nearly everything you know about nutrition, food, and your body has been taught by food marketers interested in corporate profit, not your health and vitality. The resulting paradigms, the subconscious programming including the omnipresent and powerful belief that calories drive health and well-being, have by extension been put there by people who do not care a whit about you or your needs. Successful wellness depends on changing those paradigms to ones that accurately reflect how things really are. Only then will the path to doing things as they ought to be done open to you.

Chapter Thirteen
Normalizing Obesity and "Diseases of Civilization"

Just this morning a client told me, "I can't wait to eat normal food again!" One of the first steps of the Nutri-90 process is to stop eating ultra-processed foods. If you remember the Lego analogy, processed foods are the sticks, stones, and little bits of unrecognizable garbage that prevent your metabolism from working properly. And yet somehow, this chemical cesspool called processed food, made in factories, stuff that was not even a thing as little as 60 years ago, is now called "normal."

Claire LaZebnik's perfect quote from her book *Epic Fail* seems apropos: "Normalcy is a lie invented by advertising agencies to make the rest of us feel inferior." It was perfect because my client was not actually craving garbage foods, but was instead just feeling out of place. She is a college student and was wanting to eat "normal food *like everyone else*."

Have you ever felt that way? Have you been to a party and felt pressure to eat whatever the host or hostess handed to you, even if you knew you shouldn't? Have you been in a restaurant or room full of people eating some sort of processed goo and felt unspoken peer pressure to join in, or even been teased by someone because of your "diet" or restrictions?

Still others feel entitled to eat whatever sort of stuff they want to eat, processed or not. A client once told me, "I can eat whatever I want. Why don't you just tell me to eat what I want, but use moderation and balance it in with what you say to eat?" Well, because to say "it is okay to eat anything so long as you use moderation" is akin to saying it is okay to hold a revolver to your head so long as five chambers are empty and only one contains a bullet. It is only a matter of time until you pull the trigger on the wrong chamber and suffer decades of chronic debilitating illness, or even death. Processed chemical poisons do not belong in your body, moderation or not.

Ad agencies have done a first-rate job, however; people today really and truly do feel somehow inferior if they do not eat whatever lines the shelves of their local superstore or is shouted from the marquee of every fast food eatery, even if doing so is going to rob them of their vitality, their mobility, and their very health and well-being. Getting fat is only the beginning; failure of the body to function is the inevitability.

The eventuality most people fear the most—loss of vitality and mobility—is the inevitable result of following the path they most fear to reject: the path of perceived normalcy.

Normalizing obesity and so-called diseases of civilization, that is to say the plethora of disease and dysfunction that stems directly from consumer choices of food, drink, and cosmetics, is absolutely the goal of marketers. It has to be; no one would continue to willingly poison themselves with cheap chemical garbage without the inherent peer pressure that accompanies perceived normalcy. It is called *social proofing*, and it is the most effective weapon in all of advertising. Put a product into enough hands and the perception will become "everyone has it; it is normal; I am deprived if I do not have it, too." And it is exactly *that*, the feeling that one is deprived somehow, that closes the deal, for we are simply not willing to feel deprived and marketers know it.

In this case, marketers are not alone. Our governmental agencies and entities must also seek to normalize obesity and disease. There is too much money flowing through the coffers to legislate against the Big Three: food & beverage, pharmaceuticals, and health care. All three profit obscenely from your sickness and immobility, and they hold the largest and strongest lobbies in the nation's capital and the capitals of every state therein. Yet in order to allow the poisoning of its citizens to continue, the government has to portray the deplorable state of our personal health as "normal."

Today you see celebrities not only accepting obesity, but celebrating it. The government is providing ever-increasing amounts of money for it. Health and pharmaceutical agencies are saying they are the only answer to it. Makers of everything from clothing to cars are adding product lines to make it attractive, comfortable, and... normal.

There is a balance to strike and I want to be very clear on this: no one should be made to suffer judgment based on their appearance. However, neither should we accept a condition that causes chronic illness and death as normal. In the same way that we readily accept a cancer patient who has lost their hair, breasts, or mobility as brave, loving them unconditionally even as they fight the cancer robbing them of their well-being, so we should approach obesity. Obesity is not normal. Obesity robs people of their vitality, their mobility, their health, their well-being, and worse, their self-esteem and sense of worth. We ought to love the brave individuals who stand up against it, and fight alongside them to conquer it and restore their health.

Calories and the Normalizing of Sickness

The calorie has been the very best tool for normalizing obesity and its related maladies. By means of the calorie, focus is diverted away from the ingredients and factory modification of food and toward moderation and personal responsibility. Now I am normally a strong advocate of personal responsibility; however, in this case it is smoke and mirrors, making you feel accountable for specific, targeted manufacturing processes, marketing, and delivery methods that are making you highly addicted to toxic substances in food, substances that are making you sick without your knowledge or permission.

In the Lego scenario I used when teaching about metabolism, I showed you that the primary function of metabolism is to disassemble food into its most basic components and then reassemble those components into all of the various molecules and cells needed by your body in the performance of myriad functions that keep you alive and thriving. When the biologically required food components are missing and have been replaced with toxic chemicals and fillers, your body does its job the best it can, but it has been handicapped in its efforts. Your body cannot keep you healthy and vital under those conditions. Food companies have altered and poisoned the food supply knowingly and, in this context, bear responsibility.

In their concerted effort to avoid responsibility, however, food companies throw calories at you. They tell you all foods are okay if you would just exercise a little moderation. They tell you your metabolism runs on calories and if you would only balance your calories-in verses your calories-out you would be healthy and fit. By keeping your attention riveted to calories, the subconscious, and very effective, message is that it doesn't matter what you eat; it only matters that you keep your calories controlled. It follows that you can eat as much of whatever that you want because you can choose to balance calories via exercise rather than portion control if you wish.

Think about this carefully, now; this is the perfect scenario for the industry and at the very same time the perfect storm for the destruction of your health and vitality:

If you focus attention on the Legos, the blame for the exponential rise of obesity and diseases of civilization fall directly at the feet of food makers, marketers, and lawmakers who pave the way for their continued existence via the wholesale lack of nutrition in their food products.

– However –

If you focus attention on calories, all blame falls directly at the feet of each individual for not exercising the simple self-control to eat less and exercise more.

Does this help you to understand why calories are the central theme of all things food and beverage? Calories are not a thing in your body and they never have been. Calories are a thing in your *mind*, and from there they deliver your personal power into the hands of industry. Like a puppet, industry can then pull the strings of power to transfer your money to their pockets in the name of being "normal."

Words Mean Things

This idea that words mean things is becoming a central theme of this book. If you have opened your mind to understand what calories really are and that they have absolutely no bearing on your metabolism, health, and well-being, then you are already on your way to freedom; the freedom to understand and apply to yourself what comes next. The entire western world has allowed this word—calorie—to be redefined by food makers, marketers, health providers, and the government, and in so doing people have abdicated their personal power into the greedy hands of those who readily and handily place their profit above your health every single time.

As long as you are willing to believe the phony definition of calorie you have been handed, and as long as you are willing to believe the calorie has anything to do with your health and well-being, that is exactly how long the industry will control you and you will be directly in harm's way, subject to every disease of civilization.

Look, I know it can be challenging to stand up against *normal*. But that challenge extends only so far as you are willing to accept another person's definition of normal.

> *"But if thought corrupts language, language can also corrupt thought."*
>
> - George Orwell, 1984

It has been said that the person who defines the words has ultimate power. You have seen how the intentional manipulation of the meaning of one word—calorie—by a profit-driven industry has manipulated an entire society into corruption of thought, action, and outcome. Don't allow it to define *your* normal. From this day forward, make it your personal determination to be in control of your own vitality, your health and well-being, your weight. Let's change the course of our discussion to that of empowerment; just how does one take action on behalf of their own wellness?

SECTION IV

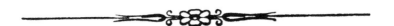

"I don't believe in the word 'incurable.' I believe to find a cure we need to deconstruct the cause."

Nikki Rowe

"No matter how much it gets abused, the body can restore balance. The first rule is to stop interfering with nature."

Deepak Chopra

Chapter Fourteen
Integrity

Please understand and believe two things at this point:

1 - The more *products* that become available, the fatter, sicker, and less vital our society becomes.
2 - The more effort expended fighting *calories*, the fatter, sicker, and less vital our society becomes.

Clearly, buying products and fighting calories has not been working. Up until this point, I have dedicated this book to helping you understand why that is true; I have been deconstructing the cause.

It saddens me to the depths of my soul every time I read a book that seems full of integrity and empowerment on the surface but turns out instead to be full of the same old bull, just pushing another product.

I want to make something really, really clear right now:

Real food, the kind that grows on farms, is for people to eat. Products—be they pills, powders, shakes, elixirs, or processed foods—are for corporate profit. There are no exceptions. Ever.

No matter what pseudoscience is used to support it, no matter how reasonable it sounds, if a speaker, book, or program ends with a sales pitch for some new supplement or other magic weight loss product, reject it and leave. No matter how impressive it looks, it is more of the same profit-driven nonsense that has brought only increased desperation and sickness. Look only for programs or information that teach you how to use real, honest food, the way society did before the so-called diseases of civilization started escalating seemingly unchecked.

As little as 60 years ago, there was no obesity epidemic. Yes, there were obese individuals, but it was not the norm. The diseases of civilization, including obesity and its complications, are self-made. We have collectively allowed ourselves to be educated about food by marketers, and this world of uncontrolled weight gain and sickness is the end game.

Neither I nor my company are involved in selling processed products of any kind, including foods and supplements. We are solely guided by the empowerment of people to become champions of their own wellness and well-being, including weight loss.

Now is the time for *your* empowerment. Are you ready?

Chapter Fifteen
Vitality, Wellness, and
the Zen of Food

Math is often referred to as the universal language because it never varies, no matter where you are in the world or universe. Algebra in America will have the same solutions as algebra in Russia or Japan. Calculations made in Texas will still work on the moon or on Mars.

In algebra, we learn about variables and how to solve for them. If we follow the rules of algebra, we are led to a solution. We will reach the same solution regardless of where we are in the world, and others can use our solution and build on it in their own work. There is a caveat here, then; if we err in our calculations and compute an incorrect variable, everything that builds upon that variable will also be incorrect.

It is not a surprise that math is employed in every field of science because of its universal nature and precise structure. Now here is something that every true scientist knows: when a premise, or hypothesis, is accurate, the math will prove it out. If the math does not work, there is something wrong with the hypothesis, or at least something missing.

In this book, we have used a similar process to prove that calories are not a thing in the human body. Calorie math does not work. Those who profit from the idea of calories are putting forth ever more convoluted math and increasingly confusing explanations while trying desperately to hold onto a premise that simply does not compute.

Now that we have proved the point, let's drop math and science and focus instead on something much simpler. In the days of our grandparents and great-grandparents, folks understood matters of food and health. Their understanding did not come to them by means of science or complicated reasoning; they just knew. There was a collective consciousness about food and wellness that sprouted and matured from the thousands of years that people and food have coexisted. This thing worked and that thing didn't, and that information was passed from generation to generation.

At Nutri-90, we call that the Zen of Food, or a phrase of our own coinage, *Shiwu Zen*. Now don't attack me for my poor use and translation of Chinese; that would miss the point. Shiwu Zen very loosely translates as "the Zen of food." And *that* is the point.

Taken outside of the spiritual context, Zen means "an approach to an activity, skill, or subject that emphasizes simplicity and intuition rather than conventional thinking or fixation on goals."[34] Or, as another source suggests, being "relaxed and not worrying about things that you cannot change."[35]

We have created a society that, by and large, dismisses intuition in favor of that which is perceived as science and "fact." Very often, though, as we have proven, fact is not fact at all, and neither is it science; rather, it is the workings of a profit-driven machine bent on controlling your mind and emotions in order to line its pockets with your money.

When people simply *understood* food and wellness intuitively, we were a healthier, fitter population than we are today, by a wide margin. Someone always wants to argue this point with me, pulling out some statistic or another. But this fact remains true and indisputable: as processed convenience foods, supplements, medicines, meal replacement shakes and bars, "adult nutrition" food aisles in

115

supermarkets, self-styled "nutrition centers," and "wellness centers" proliferate, the health of America's citizens is going straight down the drain. So much so, in fact, that the average American has lost some or all of their vitality and mobility by age 50, often much sooner than that.[36]

So let's take a look at food from the perspective of Shiwu Zen, the easy, effective path to that elusive goal we all seek: vitality, wellness, fitness, and total body health. There are three aspects to this discussion:
1. the center of your focus,
2. the placement of your emotions, and
3. the balance of your food.

Ready? Let's go!

Chapter Sixteen
Shiwu Zen:
The Center of Focus

Where you place your focus is important to the quality of your outcomes. Let me give an example: a person who focuses solely on making more money is likely to lose integrity eventually, because they will make desperate decisions sooner or later in the quest to achieve their focus. No amount of money will satiate them. However, a person who focuses on providing *value* to their clients will maintain their integrity, and most likely make more than enough money in the process. Both people want to live well; however, the person who focused on the path before them in addition to the destination is less likely to get tripped up and fall. The first person must always chase money, while the second person, because they provided a value that others will seek, finds money chasing them!

Have you ever heard someone say they were never successful in love until they stopped trying to find someone? Then, magically, a great partner appeared. It is the same principle; instead of always focusing on their next partner, a person focused on bettering themselves will find partners chasing the better person they have become.

In the world of wellness, most folks these days are chasing weight loss. Just like the person chasing money, they find that weight comes and goes; they can never lose enough and it always comes back, and they become more and more desperate. They then find themselves trying more and more desperate solutions. Have you experienced this cycle of frustration, desperately trying but achieving little or no permanent success? If you slow down and let yourself reflect on the reasons for your struggles, you will realize your focus is in the wrong place.

Most people see wellness in a hierarchical fashion with weight at the top, like this:

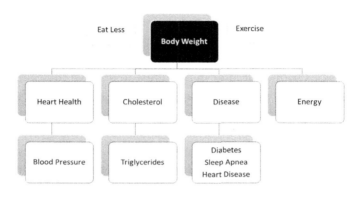

MOST PEOPLE SEE WELLNESS IN A HIERARCHICAL FASHION

This view of wellness derives from the CICO model. Remember, CICO means "calories-in-calories-out." This model holds that diseases of civilization are caused by obesity and being overweight, and that the path to freeing yourself from disease is to lose weight. Has your doctor ever told you that you must lose weight in order to bring your blood pressure down, reduce your cholesterol, or lower your risk of diabetes or heart disease? If you are overweight or obese, you have very likely heard something like that at a recent doctor visit.

Following the CICO model, your focus would be squarely on weight loss and, it would logically follow, your path to success would be to eat less and exercise more, a path designed to burn more calories while eating less of them. Now that you know calories are not a thing in the human body, you understand why the CICO model can lead only to frustrated efforts and eventual failure. So what model does work? What point of focus leads to success, not only with weight loss but with overall wellness, every time? How can you plan and take action to achieve the real goals of vitality, mobility, and fitness?

Do you remember the Lego analogy from Chapter Five? Just a quick review will help you identify the exact point of focus which leads to improved wellness, including weight loss. Like the person who gains money by focusing on providing value to clients, you will see surprisingly quick and effective weight loss, along with all sorts of other health and vitality benefits, by focusing on that part of you which is responsible for managing your Legos.

Your focus must be on your *metabolism*. Catabolism disassembles larger molecules, such as your food, into their smallest usable parts and pieces, like a child taking apart a Lego project into its smallest individual blocks. Anabolism reassembles those parts and pieces into larger molecules that your body then uses to build itself, maintain itself, heal itself, and perform the myriad other functions required by life. These two functions, taken together, are your metabolism. Remember: ***metabolism is why life exists***. Without it, there would be no life of any kind anywhere in the universe. It is the most beautiful system of systems which has ever come into being, worthy of admiration, respect, and the utmost care.

By extension, then, ***caring for your metabolism and giving it the raw materials it requires is essential to your existence, and the quality of the raw materials you provide will directly affect the quality of your existence***. I want you to remember this one point above all others.

Understanding that your metabolism is the center of health, wellness, and vitality allows you to redirect your focus away from weight loss and toward your metabolism. By extension, you will also be caring for every aspect of your body, mind, and soul.

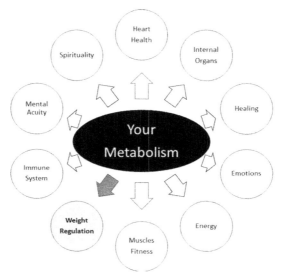

WELLNESS SEEN HOLISTICALLY

The nutrients you feed your metabolism are utilized in the creation, constant healing, and regeneration of the physical *you*. But it does not stop there, not by a long shot. The nutrients you feed your metabolism are used to create and regenerate the neurocircuits used to map your memories; the receptors and transmitters used in inter-cellular communication; the hormones and receptors used to elicit emotion; and so much more. Quite literally, everything that makes you *you* is a direct result of metabolic activity, and that activity is limited only by the quality of the raw materials you provide via the consumer choices you make for yourself each day.

Do you remember in Chapter Twelve when we discussed paradigms and the myriad subconscious decisions you make every day? Your choice of focus is a controlling paradigm; that is to say it is an overriding directive that instantly affects your other subconscious programs. Let's say, for example, you really want a new TV and you focus your desire on a specific make and model. Your other internal paradigms, or programs, will follow suit as you begin to save to purchase the TV, willingly work overtime for it, prioritize it above other purchases, and so on. You will almost certainly bend heaven and earth to make that purchase happen and see the TV in your living room.

By the same mechanism, your daily choices and decisions will inexorably be shifted, in all manner of ways, if you make just one conscious choice: take your focus *off* weight loss and put it *on* proper nutrition for your metabolism.

That is really hard for some people, and it may be really hard for you. Everything about our social consciousness is wrapped up in beach bodies, sexual desirability, and Hollywood notions of femininity and masculinity as physical attributes rather than facets of character. It may be challenging to break away from the daily desire to lose pounds. But I tell you this truly: weight loss becomes much, much more productive, easier, and sustainable once you stop focusing on it. That may sound counterintuitive, but it is absolutely true for the simple reason that by shifting focus to metabolic nourishment, you are shifting focus into harmony with how your body really works. And that makes every difference in the world.

Chapter Seventeen
Shiwu Zen:
The Placement of Emotion

Closely related to choosing your point of focus is the proper placement of your emotions. There is a school of thought which asserts that you have no control over your emotions; they just happen and you have to deal with them as they occur. That is true of some emotions, yes. If a loved one dies, for instance, you must allow the grieving process to happen, including the flood of heavy emotions. But other emotions occur because of your thoughts and the way you see the world, and you have the power to change that.

Zen philosophy involves dropping illusion and seeing things without the distortion created by your own thoughts. Do you remember the definition of common sense I chose to begin Section II? The first part of that definition was this: "Common sense is the knack of seeing things as they are…." Doesn't that sound a lot like Zen? Look at the two this way:

"Seeing things without the distortion created by your own thoughts"

"The knack of seeing things as they [really] are"

Wow. Zen is really common sense. Common sense *is* Zen. *{poof}* Mind blown.

Emotions are, in large part, orchestrated by your perception of the world. Your emotions can be altered, therefore, if your perception of the world changes.

In his book *The 7 Habits of Highly Effective People*, Dr. Steven Covey gave a fantastic illustration on just this topic, which I paraphrase here:[37]

> A man on a train was distracted, and inattentive to his children. His children were behaving in a rude manner: thumping on the back of newspapers being read by fellow travelers, running in the aisles, and being loud and unruly.
>
> One fellow traveler became more and more agitated, until finally his anger rose to the surface. He understandably felt that the father of these children should take control and care for his children, and discipline them so they would stop causing so many problems for the others on the train.
>
> This traveler took action and approached the father of the children. "Why won't you take charge of your kids? They are disrupting everyone else on the train while you just sit there, doing nothing!"
>
> The father looked around, seemingly noticing his children and the disruption on the train for the first time. The fellow traveler noticed as the father looked up that his eyes were wet, and tears had been streaming down his face.
>
> "Oh, I am so very sorry," the father said. "The kids' mom died earlier this afternoon. I can't seem to focus…. I am so sorry."
>
> The father gathered his children to him and hugged them. The fellow traveler returned to his seat, no longer full of anger. Instead, his heart was full of compassion, and he helped other passengers

understand what had happened so they, too, would feel supportive rather than agitated.

Do you see how changing your view of the world automatically changes everything else along with it, including your emotions and actions?

Attaching emotion to the reading on a bathroom scale emanates from a misdirected, or perhaps misinformed, perception of the world. Listen to Zen, or common sense, for a moment: the number on your scale is a data point. It is an important data point, but it is nevertheless only data, only information.

You work with data every day. Would you want to make important decisions in your life without the best data, or information, available? Of course not! Business owners spend huge amounts of money on data systems that keep decision-making information at their fingertips.

Data. Information to use when making your next decision. That's all the number on a scale is.

When people step on scales, though, they are ecstatic if numbers drop, and often depressed or discouraged if numbers rise: a vast range of emotions. Why?

Simply put, it is because, in that person's current view of the world, the number on their scale represents success or failure. But those numbers have nothing to do with real success or failure. They are data points. *Success or failure will come from what choice they make next—not the data itself, but the decisions made using that data*. Strong emotion will most assuredly skew the next decision that person makes, though, and likely not for the better. Ecstatic happiness at a good number causes folks to make poor food decisions in "celebration." Shame, discouragement, and depression cause folks to make poor food choices seeking "comfort food." Tying emotions to scale numbers is a lose-lose proposition for you. It is data, and should be viewed from a more clinical perspective, devoid of emotional entanglement.

In the 1920s, American society twisted calories into a moral statement. Gaining weight meant you were eating too many calories, and that was seen as "cheating" on the part of the "offender." Since eating less calories than you burned was such a simple concept to grasp, there was no "excuse" for not following it personally. And so an entire system of interpersonal judgmentalism was born, and negative people were quick to begin using it.

If you have carefully considered what you have been reading thus far, you are now on your way to *intellectual freedom* from the burden of the calorie lie. The only thing standing between your intellectual freedom and your *emotional freedom* is acceptance. Accept that the information you have learned is true, and your emotions will follow. Judging yourself by numbers on a scale will suddenly seem counterproductive.

Take another look at the image on page 120. Look at it carefully, then come back to this page....

What did you see in that image? You saw that your metabolism is responsible for everything that is life. To function optimally on *any* level, your metabolism must be provided what it needs for *all* levels. If you deliver that by following the guidelines in this section, then your metabolism will take the next step by prioritizing its many and varied responsibilities efficiently and effectively.

Weight regulation is one of those responsibilities, but it is not the only responsibility; you see that, right? Your metabolism does not actually want you to have excess body weight. We will address that shortly; for now, realize and accept that your metabolism will throw that unnecessary fat away as soon as you provide an environment that allows that process to commence. At the same time, you must accept that weight loss might not always be the highest priority. If you have an invading virus, as one example, your metabolism will see to that first. Keeping you alive is job number one, and eliminating the invading virus is more important at that moment. Extreme stress can affect several systems managed by your metabolism, and as such may also be prioritized. Severe physical trauma that requires repair and regeneration can take priority over weight loss. Weight loss will most definitely happen; you must trust your metabolism to make it happen at the right time and at the correct priority level.

Take a moment and think: if you were responsible for keeping someone alive, how would you prioritize the many tasks involved? How would you choose to use your available resources for that person's best interests? There is a very good chance your metabolism will prioritize in the same way that you would.

If you genuinely grasp and appreciate this simple idea—that your metabolism beautifully and perfectly prioritizes every task necessary to keep you alive and thriving—the number on the scale jumps into perspective, doesn't it? My clients are constantly amazed when I suggest that they may have an infection or low-grade illness, and a few days later the symptoms hit them. In rare cases clients have seemingly stalled on the scale for weeks, and then learned they had a more serious medical issue beneath the surface. Am I somehow prescient? Can I foresee the future? No, not at all! I simply understand that which I just shared with you. If you properly provide for your metabolism and your scale is not showing any loss of your excess weight, there can be only one reason: your metabolism has prioritized something else as more important. Maybe you have an illness; perhaps you are experiencing greater than normal stress; you may be sleep deprived. Whatever it is, don't feel depressed or discouraged by your scale number but instead rejoice, because your metabolism is working! It is caring for you! It is keeping you alive!

If you follow this logic, you have to ask me now: how is it that you have gained so much excess weight in the first place, even though some of that weight, the visceral weight, can be so dangerous to your health and well-being? The answer is the same: your metabolism has prioritized something more important. *Gaining* excess weight is a sign that, in all probability, you have poisoned your body with so many toxic food choices that your metabolism has placed itself in *crisis mode*.

You may have heard the term "crisis mode" before. This is a very real metabolic phenomenon; however, it has been mistakenly cast as a function of calorie deficiency. Now that you can discern that calories are not a thing in the human body and that your metabolism does not burn anything at all, you are free to understand and accept that crisis mode is your metabolism's answer to an entirely different deficiency.

I want you to pretend for a moment. Pretend you are the captain of a submarine in the center of a very large and deep ocean. Your engines have stopped and you have experienced catastrophic power failure. Your submarine has sunk to the bottom of the sea and you only have minimal backup power. You do not yet know what has caused the failures, and help is far away. What will you do first?

I am sure you can imagine how terrifying this scenario would be, and there are a lot of tasks that would need to be completed in short succession if you hope to survive it. As the captain, you understand the sudden dramatic increase in the value of your available resources. One of your first actions, then, will be to lock up all of those resources, including your food, drinking water, and anything else that will need to be rationed. There will be two keys to the locked areas; you will keep one and give the other to someone you trust implicitly, and both keys will be necessary to access any of the locked-up materials. Those resources will then be rationed in the smallest amounts possible that allow your crew to work on the problems at hand, and to hopefully repair the affected systems and get your boat back in motion.[*]

Why would you take that action? Because human nature would otherwise lead almost every member of your crew to horde those resources as soon as the reality of the crisis sank into their consciousness. They would horde more resources than they required for the purpose of keeping themselves alive as long as possible. That is a basic survival instinct which is common to all human beings. Because of it, you would find your food, water, and other necessities depleted almost immediately, just as you see stores on the news looted and emptied in the face of natural disasters.

Your metabolism has a similar primal function: first and foremost, its job is to keep you alive. The quality of that life will depend on the quality of the resources your metabolism receives. If the resources received are of poor quality and largely unusable, your metabolism will horde everything it does receive until it finds what it needs to fix you and to begin functioning properly. Even worse, if the resources received

---

[*] The author understands the deviations between this illustration and actual Navy procedures. Please tolerate the license for clarity in teaching how the body works.

by your metabolism are, in fact, toxic and they leech away nutrients desperately needed by your body, your metabolism will horde more still.

This horded material is your body fat. It is there for one reason only: you are *malnourished*. You are not putting the nutrients into your body that it desperately requires. Your metabolism is in crisis mode.

You may not immediately accept this notion of malnourishment and metabolic crisis mode in the face of excess weight. How could you possibly be malnourished when you are clearly eating more than enough? Ahhh, there it is again: calorie thinking. This is not about calories, remember? You could eat all of the food in Aisle 4 and still be malnourished if your metabolism has received toxic levels of poisonous chemicals and inadequate amounts of the 90+ nutrients it actually needs. There is a name for this: we call it *overfed-undernourished*. It is often described as the *obesity paradox*.*

So, if you have chosen foods that place your metabolism in a state of crisis and it hordes resources, causing your scale to move upward, does it make sense to feel depressed or discouraged? No, not at all. That would be like giving a child water and bricks and being disappointed they could not start a fire. The scale gives data; it is providing you the information you can use to begin making better decisions for yourself. You may never have realized this before, but now you have the missing piece that has prevented your understanding. Now you know what your metabolism is telling you. Now you are learning what to do.

---

* The term "obesity paradox" is also used in reference to certain relationships between weight and heart attack survival rates. That is a different discussion, and not our purpose here.

Emotion is a powerful force that will cause you either to act in your own best interests or to self-destruct. The difference lies in how you perceive the world around you. Stop deadening every communication your body sends to you and instead listen to it: perceive what it is telling you. Pain, soreness, itchiness, discomfort, even that number on your scale—it all means something. Don't take pills to make those symptoms go away; listen to them and adjust your decisions accordingly.

Trust that your body is making decisions that are in your very best interest. That one modification alone—trusting your own body—can change everything about the placement of your emotions. Stop blaming genetics, your thyroid, metabolic dysfunction, or whatever new fad buzzword is in the media today. This is about what you choose to put into your body. Period. So love that body! Give it some respect! Cherish it! Your body is beautiful, and it will always do its very best to keep you alive and thriving, vital, excited, and enthused. Obesity is nothing more than you getting in its way. Trust this, friend; I was right there with you once. I know.

So you have adjusted your focus away from calories and toward nutrients. You have moved your emotions away from judgmentalism and justification and toward loving your very special hardworking body and its metabolism. Now what? What do you *do* to lose that weight, optimize your heath, and finally realize that oh-so-elusive vitality and quality of life?

Chapter Eighteen
Shiwu Zen:
The Balance of Food

This is what everyone wants to know about. This is the burning question my new clients can't wait to ask. You may even have fast-forwarded to this chapter because you can't wait to know the secret, too. This is the Holy Grail of the entire book, after all.

What do I eat to lose weight?
What do I eat to be healthier?
Where are the recipes?

Listen. If you haven't done so already, please back up and read this book from the start before diving into this chapter. There is an unchangeable law in the universe that goes like this:

Your beliefs directly determine your outcomes.

It is true. The information contained in this chapter has the power to change everything for you. It can open the door for you to easily:

- Lose weight
- Regain vitality
- Lower blood pressure
- Normalize cholesterol and triglycerides
- Optimize your metabolism
- Empower yourself to gain control over your own life

But only if you believe it. And you will only believe it if you understand how your metabolism works and why it is the very center of every facet of your existence. I have every confidence that, by reading this book from the start, you will understand. When you understand, you will believe. When you believe, this chapter will give you the tools to change your outcomes.

As Americans, we want to believe we are free. I hear clients every day tell me they desire freedom: the freedom to eat or drink anything they wish, whenever they wish it. Do you feel that way? If you do, you should consider closely what you know about alcoholics and drug addicts. Modern, processed convenience foods do not represent freedom. They embody slavery: slavery to food addictions engineered by corporations for the sole purpose of transferring your personal power to their executives, and your money to their pockets. That's it. Slavery. If you don't believe me, try eliminating all processed convenience foods from your diet. Then, when the "cravings" strike so hard that you just *have* to eat more to get your next fix, explain to me how you are *free* to choose. If you cannot choose health without such powerful addictive responses, then freedom is not yours for the taking. You can only be truly free if you are free from slavery to *anything* which would control you, and that includes slavery to food addictions. Let's get free right now.

The Story So Far

Thus far, we have set the stage for what is to come.

You have learned exactly what your metabolism is, what it does, and how it does it. In so learning, you have discovered the workings of catabolism and anabolism and uncovered a little-known truth: that your metabolism does not "burn" anything.

You have lifted the veil from the most ubiquitous, universally accepted lie in recent history—the calorie—and proven it is not a thing at all in your body.

You have exposed the primary tactic of food marketers—classical conditioning—and revealed how marketers have used this simple technique to tie food to every event you attend, every place you go, and every emotion you feel, creating a "one meal per day" environment in which people are literally eating or drinking something all day long.

You have discovered how to recognize your deep-seated beliefs—your paradigms—and, upon realizing you had little to do with their creation, you have learned how to take control of them and reprogram them for yourself.

You have examined current social efforts to normalize obesity and the diseases of civilization, and seen why those efforts feed corporate profit while relegating you to a life of chronic illness and maybe even premature death.

Having read and reflected upon these important topics, are you ready to assume responsibility for your own health, vitality, wellness, and longevity? Are you ready to become *empowered* to take charge of your own wellness?

The Three Disciplines of Shiwu Zen

The mechanics of Shiwu Zen are really quite straightforward and simple. The only challenges come from one's own focus and emotions. Following the counsel throughout this book will help you overcome those challenges, and the coaches of Nutri-90 stand ready to help if you want or need additional support.

The Three Disciplines of Shiwu Zen are these:

1. **Drink the correct amount of water every day.**
2. **Eliminate consumption of any product that contains toxic substances which block your metabolism from fully fulfilling its functions.**
3. **Balance the types of food you eat each day in proportion to your metabolism's needs for specific nutrient groups.**

It really is that simple. We will explore each discipline individually, and you will readily recall the details later simply by memorizing these three bullets verbatim.

A mentor once told me, "Belldon, Nike said it right. Just do this stuff." I pass the same advice on to you: just do this stuff. If you commit just 30 days to following the details of this chapter implicitly, you will *feel* the difference. You will *see* the difference. You will *experience* the difference. Your personal success will robustly motivate you to continue down the path of your own empowerment.

A few cautions as we begin:

First, you may know people who are clients of Nutri-90, people who have lost seemingly incredible amounts of weight and have seen tremendous improvements in their health and quality of life. Tony in Santa Cruz, for example, lost 231 pounds in sixteen months, reversed his sleep apnea, and normalized his cholesterol and blood pressure. Anna in Houston lost 128 pounds in twelve months and reversed her prediabetes diagnoses. Vicki in Seattle lost 27 pounds she had not been able to lose in more than two decades of effort, and learned how to manage weight while living with Hashimoto's Disease. The momentum of her success opened doors to fulfilling many additional personal goals. Donna in California has, at the time of this writing, lost 149 pounds in nine months and is well on her way to her optimum weight. She has already regained much of her mobility and changed the course of her future. Carrie in Washington, at age 71, lost 48 pounds and stabilized her blood pressure and cholesterol. For the first time in more than 30 years, her doctor took her off of her heart medicines. Karina in California lost 43 pounds as a teenager in junior high school.

Every one of these real people[*] has kept their weight off, some for many years. However, you should know that these people and thousands of others like them are one-to-one clients of Nutri-90 and have received daily personal attention along with personalized program design and strategies. Don't judge your progress compared to these, or any other, clients. Your metabolism will progress at the pace that is right for you.

By following what you are about to learn, you will improve your health, your vitality, and your quality of life for the better, likely in dramatic ways, and you can and will lose unwanted pounds. At the same time, you must realize that every person is unique and has their own health issues, their own lifestyle, their own allergies, and myriad other traits that affect their optimal metabolic nutrient profile. You also have *your* own unique individual profile. Don't judge your progress against the stories you have heard from others who may be receiving personal, one-to-one attention. Instead, evaluate your progress by how you feel compared to last week and revel in the improvements.

Acknowledge and embrace your personal development and progress. Don't be afraid to love yourself for it.

---

[*] Some names have been changed by request of the clients.

Second, remember what you have learned and trust your body. If you are primarily looking for weight loss, you have to understand this:

Weight loss does not automatically lead to wellness, but wellness does *lead to weight loss.*

Shiwu Zen does not seek to force weight loss, but instead seeks to provide nourishment for your metabolism. Your metabolism, in turn, cares for every aspect of your body, mind, and spirit, and the process of nourishing it causes a rate of weight loss that surprises most people. If your scale does not seem to cooperate for a couple of days, trust that your metabolism is prioritizing its many responsibilities exactly as it is designed to do; it will get back to weight loss at exactly the right time for it. Whatever your metabolism is caring for at a given moment is essential to your health and well-being, and eating the balance of foods you will learn about shortly is the very best path to support your metabolism in its efforts. Weight loss will come in its time; if you are patient, you will find it really does happen much faster than you might imagine.

Okay—are you ready to get your Zen on?

DISCIPLINE 1 - WATER

Hydration is the most important component your body needs, and it is maybe the most overlooked by the general public. Most clients coming into Nutri-90 drink between one and five glasses of water per day. That is just terrible!

Between 55 and 60 percent of your body is water. Take just a moment and do the math on that. How much do you weigh? Divide that number by two. The resulting number represents slightly less than the amount of water in your body. That means if you weigh 200 pounds, more than 100 of those pounds are water!

The water in your body performs more tasks than we could discuss in a book this size. Some of them include:
- Flushing toxins out of your body
- Dissolving vitamins and minerals for use by your metabolism
- Maintaining joint health
- Cushioning vital organs
- Supporting cellular vitality
- Preserving youthful, vibrant skin

Water is—really is—the elixir of life. Your body tells you so, too. Just become dehydrated and listen to your body scream: intense headaches, dizziness, nausea, and even fainting may occur depending on your level of dehydration.

One hundred pounds of water is a little more than eleven gallons. Do you really suppose that drinking five cups per day is adequate to keep your body's water refreshed?

There is no consensus at all in nutritional and scientific circles about how much water is enough. Decades ago, someone decided that drinking eight 8-ounce glasses was a good standard: 64 ounces per day. The Institute of Medicine has set a higher standard: nine glasses per day for women and thirteen for men.

Two things are universal in almost all standards, though: the standards treat all people as though they are the same, and the standards treat almost all liquids as though they are the same. Both of those suppositions are false.

To assume a 4-foot, 11-inch women weighing 105 pounds requires exactly the same daily water intake as my good friend Sam, who stands 6-foot 2-inches and weighs 265 pounds, is absurd. Her body might contain 58 pounds of water while his may contain 160 pounds of water, almost three times more! Clearly they should be drinking different amounts, wouldn't you say?

The other universal commonality of popular hydration advice is equally illogical. The belief that all liquids count toward daily hydration requirements is pushed hard, especially by soda makers. Coca-Cola executive Katie Bayne once said in an interview, "What our drinks offer is hydration. That's essential to the human body. We offer great taste and benefits.... We don't believe in empty calories. We believe in hydration."[38] Nothing could be further from reality.

Here is the truth. Liquids contain water, but that water is not always usable by your body. Drinks like alcohol, coffee, tea, soda, and even some bottled mineral waters are diuretic, meaning they actually cause free water to release from the body and be eliminated. That is not always a bad thing, but your body also needs water it can circulate and use. In this capacity, only water is water. And only pure water is free of extraneous ingredients that are potentially harmful to you.

While it is true that real, farm-fresh foods also contain water, that water is not easily quantifiable; the normal human has a life to lead and doesn't walk around calculating the hydration viability of each thing they eat every day. It is generally acknowledged that food provides less than 20 percent of the water required by your body. Drinking the correct amount of water for your body to thrive, then, becomes very important.

In the absence of a solid scientific answer to the question "How much water should I drink?" we turn to anecdotal evidence; what works for real people living in the real world?

Those of us who work in wellness tend to recommend the crazy-easy-to-calculate and universally effective guidance to drink one-half of your body weight in ounces of water daily. In short, if you weigh 200 pounds, drink 100 ounces of water daily; if you weigh 160 pounds, drink 80 ounces of water daily; if you weigh 300 pounds, drink 150 ounces of water daily; and so on. Given the importance of water to your metabolism, I believe it is better to err on the side of too much, rather than too little.

A lot of really cool things begin to happen when you start drinking the correct amount of water. Most of my clients see weight loss begin from just this one step. Joints feel better. Thinking is easier. You may feel more alert and energetic. Skin starts looking fresher and more youthful. Yes, water does all those things!

Coffee and tea are fine to drink, but don't count them toward your daily water amount. Remember: only water is water.

And yes, you may pee a lot when you first start drinking the right amount of water. Your body is not used to it, after all. But don't worry; that will normalize after a few days of receiving proper hydration.

Let me share one added benefit of water you might really appreciate. When you lose a lot of weight, proper water throughout the process will help tighten loose skin and keep you looking and feeling awesome. Loose skin does happen when a person loses a great deal of weight. With proper hydration from the very start of your journey, though, loose skin is minimized, and it usually tightens up over time after the weight is lost.

Here is what you want to do:

1- Divide your scale weight by two; this will be the total amount of water, in ounces, you want to drink each and every day. As you lose weight, you may also reduce your water intake according to this formula, if you wish.

2- Drink one-third of your daily amount of water before lunch. Drink the next third between lunch and dinner. Drink the final third after dinner. If you do not want to be up too often peeing at night, finish drinking your water about two hours before bedtime.

3- The best way to get your water is to buy a water filter for your home and get your filtered water from your own tap. Brita and PUR both make filters for reasonable prices that fit on your kitchen faucet.

DISCIPLINE 2 - ELIMINATE STICKS, STONES, AND BROKEN PIECES OF UNIDENTIFIABLE STUFF

I am going to be completely honest right here and now: it does little good to start eating the *right* things unless you also stop eating the *wrong* things. Modern processed foods contain all sorts of ingredients that block the passage of essential nutrients into your body and hamper your metabolism from doing its job, which is to keep you alive and thriving. It is absolutely imperative that you stop putting poison into your body.

Remember the Lego analysis. When you give a child sticks, stones, and broken pieces of unidentifiable stuff mixed in with their building blocks, it becomes impossible to build beautiful and useful things. The garbage pieces will not attach properly to the building blocks. They either cannot be used at all or, at best, will make the completed structures weak and ugly.

Garbage food works the same way in your body. Your metabolism cannot use it or, at best, can only make weak and inadequate structures. Listen, even you call it "junk food." Would you willingly put junk gas in your car? Would you give junk toys to your kids? Do you choose the junkiest tree you can find for Christmas? Not likely! So why on earth would you willingly put junk food into your body?

Remember what you learned earlier: your metabolism is the very center of everything that makes you who you are, physically, spiritually, mentally, and emotionally. Metabolism uses the raw materials you provide to create everything necessary to keep all of those aspects of your being alive and well. It follows that the quality of *you* cannot exceed the quality of the raw materials you make available to your metabolism. Think about it. This is just physics, an unchangeable law of the universe. Junk food equals junk *you*.

I am not going to list all of the foul ingredients in modern processed foods; there are already plenty of books and online sources for that. I will talk about only three of the more insidious ingredients here, and I hope that is enough for you to realize that you cannot get healthy, nor remain healthy, unless you stop putting garbage into your body. Your metabolism cannot do its job when it is inhibited by the sticks, stones, and unrecognizable pieces of broken stuff that is processed convenience food and junk food.

Calcium disodium EDTA (Ethylenediaminetetraacetic acid): This chemical is made by mixing formaldehyde, sodium cyanide, and the chelating agent ethylenediaminetetraacetic acid. It is used to keep white foods white, to keep creamy foods creamy, and to preserve things that should spoil in a week—things like mayonnaise—almost indefinitely.

Look, there is nothing good about this stuff. In fact, there is sufficient reason to be concerned about it on many levels, and even the FDA advises limiting consumption to less than three grams per day and never more than five days in a row. Consuming more than this is considered toxic to humans and has been linked to birth defects, cancer, genetic mutation, kidney disease, and even death.[39]

To me, that is sufficient reason to avoid it altogether. It is not something that belongs in or on a human body. And those limits? If you eat processed convenience or junk foods, I guarantee you are ingesting this stuff every single day. It is found in mayonnaise, creamy salad dressings, certain canned vegetables, prepared foods and meals, soda, sauces, and much more. It is also an ingredient in nearly all sunscreens, liquid bath soaps, shampoos, and conditioners, as well as a plethora of makeup products. It is becoming harder and harder to avoid.

Besides the ingredient calcium disodium EDTA, just the EDTA component is found in iron-fortified breads and cereals. You see, iron rusts when oxidized, causing discoloration and an unpleasant taste in those fortified foods. By bonding the iron with EDTA, the iron is stabilized and does not result in that perceived nastiness.

This latter use is one you should think about and understand, because it perfectly illustrates the importance of eliminating processed foods from your body as much as possible.

EDTA is a chelating agent. That means it bonds to metals, rendering them inert. It is used medicinally to treat heavy metal poisoning. Emergency room doctors will inject it into the veins of a person who is suffering heavy metal poisoning and the EDTA will bond to the metals in the bloodstream, rendering them inert, after which the body will hopefully eliminate them without further damage to the patient.

In the case of emergency room medicine, EDTA is awesome and it saves lives. However, in the case of your food, it is absolutely insane. The reason it prevents iron from tainting your food is because it bonds to the iron, rendering it inert. In that condition, iron cannot be used properly by your metabolism, either. Remember the medicinal use of EDTA? It is used to leach metals *out* of the body, *preventing their absorption*. By eating foods which contain EDTA, it stands to reason that the same thing is happening, except in the absence of toxic heavy metals the target becomes metals and minerals that are essential to your wellness, the ones that are *supposed* to be in your body.

Iron deficiency is a real problem for western women. Is it any wonder? Our food supply pretends to provide increased iron via "iron-fortified" foods, which actually leach iron and other vital nutrients out of the body instead.

Your body utilizes bio-electrical communication between cells to identify and eliminate disease and abnormality and to ensure adequate nutrition. Trace metals are essential to that process. Leaching them out of your body by the food you choose contributes to disease and deficiency in part by limiting that bioelectric communication.

All of this chaos is caused by *just one* chemical in your food supply. Processed garbage foods also contain industrial solvents, lighter fluid, petroleum distillates, known carcinogens, neuro-blockers, chemicals linked to hyperactivity and Alzheimer's disease, and the list goes on for some distance. You cannot expect health and vitality, or even sustainable weight loss, if the raw materials you provide to your metabolism include pollutants like these. Putting this poison into your body will lead to suffering in every way: physically, spiritually, mentally, and emotionally.

Do you want to know what breaks my heart and makes me cry? When I see a client whose family member is suffering from cancer, heart disease, or some other chronic illness that may even end in the death of the loved one, yet in some misguided quest for "comfort" the client turns to the exact same disease-inducing food, even eating it with uncontrolled abandon, binging on it. It is like standing on the tracks of the same speeding train that has already ruined the lives of thousands before you. How have we allowed marketing to blind us so completely that we seek comfort from death and disease by *eating* death and disease?

Flour: Modern American flour is not the stuff your great-grandma used. There was a time when wheat went to a mill, the mill ground it up, and that was flour, or more properly, *whole meal*. It would be ground and sifted to various consistencies for different purposes, but it was wheat. That is not the case anymore.

In the never-ending quest for increased profit, huge commercial bakeries are constantly seeking absolute consistency in their processes and ingredients, together with the longest shelf life possible for their ingredients. Whole meal does not provide either consistency or shelf life. Each crop of wheat has a different wheat berry profile and, once milled, whole meal must be stored in refrigeration because it begins to break down very quickly. It follows that each batch of flour made the old-fashioned way produces different results in breads and other baked products.

Beginning as early as the late 1800s, the quest for consistency in mass production led to numerous developments in the engineering of flour, until today's product scarcely resembles wheat at all. Early in the evolution of flour, as early as the 1920s, concern was being raised about the nutritive degeneration that seemed to go hand in hand with "advances" in flour milling technologies.[40]

Wheat today enters the factory and undergoes a major transformation. First the bran, which contains the fiber of the wheat berry, is stripped away and sold separately, fetching a higher price than flour alone. Then the germ is also stripped away and sold separately, thus eliminating most of the nutrients from the wheat.

What remains is the endosperm, a white-ish thing with little nutritive value. In order to create flour, the endosperm must undergo several steps of both chemical and mechanical conditioning, including as many as 15 steps of chemical bleaching and oxidation. Finally, the nutritionally bankrupt powder is "enriched" with synthesized vitamins and minerals.

The end product of today's flour manufacturing process is very low in usable nutrients. Worse, it is also highly addictive. Even worse still, it is very high in ultra-refined carbs. While carbs from nature in naturally delivered foods are readily identified by your metabolism and are utilized appropriately, the ultra-refined carbs in today's factory-processed flour (and sugar) are no longer in a natural state. Your metabolism cannot properly identify them, and they are almost immediately converted into sugars in your body, boosting your blood sugar levels too rapidly. This results in a stimulus to your brain similar to that induced by cocaine, a stimulus that is highly addictive in nature. It also creates imbalances between your blood sugars and insulin that, if repeated often, lead to type 2 diabetes.[41]

Someone will challenge me almost daily over the addictive nature of the garbage called flour in America. I will offer this thought-provoking insight: You know those things you call "carb cravings" that drive you straight to sugar and baked goods? Those absolutely are *not* cravings for carbs. If they were actually carb cravings, they would be satisfied by fruits or vegetables, which contain plenty of naturally derived carbs for your metabolism to thrive. But it isn't carbs that people crave, it is refined flour, refined sugar, or both. These aren't cravings; they are addictions.

Most folks realize by now the dangers of refined sugar. Few grasp the menace that is modern refined flour. To realize metabolic optimization, including a healthy heart, weight loss, and the avoidance of debilitating disease, Shiwu Zen avoids highly refined flour and the products made with it. This includes products made with so-called multigrain flour, whole grain flour, and similar. Why? Because FDA guidelines on product labeling are murky at best, and any flour or flour-based product, except for old-style whole wheat bread, can use those monikers even if only a small percentage of the flour is the good stuff; the remaining portion is the same addictive, toxic white goo as everything else.[42]

Hidden toxic proteins: Bad things happen when the wrong things become concentrated. Food allergies are becoming more and more common even with foods to which our ancestors exhibited no sensitivity. Food addictions are also becoming more and more common. The reason for both of these problems may be traced to factory food processing methods which deliberately concentrate certain food elements.

It is no secret that processing changes the nature of food constituents. There is nothing especially addictive about tea brewed with coca leaves, for instance. Ultra-process those leaves, though, and concentrate specific compounds therein, and you have cocaine, a highly addictive drug.

As food makers have split apart the structure of foods and played with processing methods to isolate and concentrate specific compounds, similar properties have emerged in common foods. The milk protein *casein*, for example, has been found to be highly addictive in some people. When digested, casein releases protein particles called *casomorphins*, which have a strong opioid effect.[43] If you are curious how powerful opioids are, they include morphine, oxycodone, and heroin. Powerfully addictive, one and all. You may be aware of several brand-name drugs that are opioids and have made news due to their extremely addictive properties: OxyContin, Percocet, and Vicodin, for instance.

Perhaps the best thing a food company can do when they discover something addictive in food is to concentrate it. Well, that is best for the quarterly profit sheets, at least. Casein is naturally concentrated in cheese; however, food makers have been known to add additional casein, making cheese addiction a very real thing for many people.[44] Casein has been unnaturally concentrated in other dairy products as well, including yogurt and ice cream. It bears repetition that if a food is in your home that you cannot do without, even if it seems like a real farm food, that food has likely been altered. You have developed an addiction, and for that reason alone you ought to consider eliminating that food from your eating plan.

Casein can be added to dairy products without being specifically listed on the ingredient label because it is a naturally occurring milk protein. The fact that it is concentrated to addictive levels in some dairy foods does not legally necessitate a separate ingredient listing.

Casein is found as an additive in other foods though, where it does have to be listed in the ingredients. It is found in some fast food French fries, many breads, and some brands of breakfast meats, for example. There is no good reason to add stand-alone casein to those foods except to enhance their addictive quality, which it does very well.

Other food products besides dairy employ similar techniques of isolating and concentrating specific addictive proteins. The rule of thumb is simple: if you find you cannot easily stop after just a taste of a food—be it cheese, bread, peanut butter, or anything else—but instead feel compelled to eat it by the spoonful or handful and still find you are not satisfied, you are very likely eating something that has been engineered for maximum addictiveness. Great for growing corporate profit; very bad for you. That item has been tampered with, even if it's not readily obvious on the label, and it should be avoided.

What does it all mean? We could go on for days about the myriad ways food companies are tampering with the food supply, but that really isn't necessary. You already know which foods are causing you to lose balance, which foods you are addicted to. Chances are you have even told your friends or family, "I am *so* addicted to [insert food here]." You were teasing, of course, but you were also correct in a very literal sense.

I get all sorts of crazy looks from people when they learn I have eliminated processed flour from my diet. I have not eliminated bread; however, I do buy my own wheat, mill it at home, and make my own breads from scratch. I have almost entirely eliminated dairy and many other products as well. Today it is, in many places, illegal to procure dairy that has **not** been altered. If a food causes me to behave as an addict, and many dairy items do, I eliminate it.

Nearly every client that comes to Nutri-90 has something they do not want to give up. They sometimes beg to keep it in their eating plan. I tell them all the same truth. You are an adult and can choose to put anything you wish into your body; however, you can never hope to achieve a higher plane of health and vitality, or sustainable weight loss, if you choose to subject your metabolism to sticks, stones, and unrecognizable pieces of broken stuff.

Here is what you want to do:

1. Start reading *ingredient* labels. The nutrition labels are deceiving and the face labels are often outright lies; read the ingredient labels. If the product contains stuff that does not belong in your body, put it back; get rid of it. If it does not belong in your body, don't put it there.
2. If you find you are behaving like an addict over a product or food item, do not argue with yourself over it. Just get rid of it. If you "can't not have" a thing, that is exactly the thing you ought not have.
3. As much as you can, buy foods that come from local farms. I know this is not possible for everyone, but you will be better off if you buy local foods from smaller farms to whatever degree you can.
4. Buy fresh foods, not packaged foods, as much as possible.

It is not as hard to buy fresh foods as some would have you believe. No matter what, though, the greater your effort to do so, and to whatever degree you can switch away from processed, packaged foods and toward real, from-the-farm foods, to that degree you will improve your health and well-being.

DISCIPLINE 3 - BALANCING FOOD TYPES: THE LEGO SETS

Balance. In the traditional practice of Zen, two things are essential: letting go of what does not serve you, and balancing those things that do.

Balance is an important concept in every aspect of life. You balance job and family. You balance work and play. You balance cash flow.

In June of 2013, Nik Wallenda walked a high wire across an offshoot of the Grand Canyon, a quarter mile above the canyon floor below. Balance? Oh, hell yeah.

I often use Nik's feat as an analogy of the balance of food, to illustrate the fact that "a little" and "a lot" are sometimes the same thing. If Nik lost his balance "a lot," he would be in mortal danger of falling to his death. If Nik lost his balance "a little," he would be in mortal danger of... falling to his death. There is no difference.

Is balancing food the same thing as balancing on a 2-inch wire 1,500 feet above the rocks below? No. Food kills much, much more slowly.

Shiwu Zen, or the balance of food, requires eliminating consumption of the processed toxic stuff and instead consuming a *balance* of the good stuff.

If the toxic stuff is eliminated and we are no longer eating poisonous, processed sticks, stones, and unrecognizable broken stuff, why is *balancing* healthy food choices so important? Won't we be okay just by *eating* only healthy foods?

Actually, no. Eating healthy foods is not the same as healthy eating. There are many folks these days trying to eat only healthy foods yet still missing the mark on their health and wellness goals.

Think once again of the Legos. If you provide your metabolism with the correct building blocks to work with, but only red and blue square blocks and little else, your metabolism will be limited as to what it can build using those limited raw materials. It will do its best, but if you need a cell structure which requires a block that wasn't provided, you will just be out of luck. If that cell was required to prevent the attack of a foreign virus or bacteria, you will be sick. The fault does not lie with your metabolism—it lies with you for not providing the needed blocks.

If you understand this analogy, then you are in the right frame of mind to understand the essence of *metabolic optimization*, providing the balance of food types that will consistently supply the correct type and amount of Legos, or metabolic building blocks.

Remember that the vast majority of our nutritional education has come from food marketers, not from independent science. Even many of the courses provided for up-and-coming nutritionists and dietitians are influenced by Big Food. For this reason, some of our placement of food types may surprise you. For example, you may think of dairy products primarily as a protein source, and the dairy industry has worked very hard and spent a great many advertising dollars to ensure that you do so. Yes, dairy has protein. However, we class it as a carb in Shiwu Zen. Many foods, both animal- and vegetable-based, contain protein. The same foods may also contain carbs. It has been our goal to determine the balance between the two; how does the body primarily use that food? What is the effect of that food on your metabolic activity? Then we class the food accordingly. We know—and you know—that many foods cross into multiple nutritional groups, yet it is our goal to keep this easy by placing foods into their primary category.

Once upon a time, there were no factory-processed foods, at least not the kind we see today. That time was not so long ago, either: as little as 60 years ago. Some foods were lightly processed and canned earlier for preservation during the World Wars, but most factory processing as we know it today began in the mid-1900s. It also was not so long ago that science had not yet opened up the world of cellular biology, which has illuminated how things work at a never-before-seen level.

Before factory processing began to redefine food, up until about 60 years ago, people *knew* how to eat. They knew the basic rules of healthy eating and what imbalances would cause disease or obesity. Shiwu Zen is based on the same balance that once was common knowledge. It is a return to the collective consciousness of a bygone generation, when obesity and the diseases of civilization were not a thing.

We are going to divide foods into four groups. Let's think of them as our Lego sets. Ensuring that you get the right number of building blocks from each set will ensure that you provide your metabolism with the raw materials it needs to make—and keep—you healthy.

Since all of us were taught "calories" almost from birth, you might immediately start counting them. Don't. Having read this book from the start, you know that calories are not a thing in your body. Nutrients are.

I would also caution that you do not get stuck in a food rut. A few of my clients at Nutri-90 start out eating only one kind of protein, one kind of fruit, and so on. Your metabolism becomes limited in its activity when it is given only limited food types, but flourishes when nourished by the wide variety of available choices.

Metabolic optimization will improve, sometimes dramatically, by inclusion of many different fresh foods. Each kind of real, fresh food has its own unique nutritional profile. Back to that once-upon-a-time, folks ate what was in season mostly, and preserved enough to last through the winter months. Seasonal eating provided the widest range of vitamins and minerals available along with a variety of proteins and carbs, ensuring that their metabolism had everything it could ever hope for. Even though you can get almost any kind of food you want almost anytime at your local market today, I urge you to sample the wide variety of foods available and constantly rotate what you eat. That way, you won't have to think much about specific nutrients; you will be getting everything from these four groups.

GROUP 1 - LEAFY GREENS

Well-prepared leafy greens are delicious, tantalizing, even sensuous.[*] When I was a kid, though, my mom knew only one way to cook a green vegetable, and that was to boil it until it was grey, lifeless, tasteless, and semi-gelatinous. Because of that early exposure, I was well into my thirties before I could make myself try a leafy green again. I hear similar stories from some of my clients who are convinced they will never enjoy a green vegetable. But listen, when I started learning the cooking techniques we teach at Nutri-90, I was amazed at how delicious this group of veggies can really be! And just

---

[*] Some medications interact dangerously with vitamin K, which is found in many leafy greens. Check with your doctor before adding leafy greens, especially if you take medications for blood clotting.

to prove it, I have tucked a few delicious recipes that include leafy greens into the back of this book. They are sumptuous. So delicious that you will serve them to company and they will ask for more!

Supplement pills, powders, and shakes are Big Food's feeble attempt to duplicate the rich and dense nutrition found in leafy greens. These vegetables are nature's own Power Supplement, and they are absolutely the most important thing we human beings should be eating every day. Take a look at the grouping, and then try one of the recipes in the back of the book and see if you do not agree that they are not only the healthiest thing you can eat, but also among the tastiest when prepared well.

Leafy greens are exactly what they say they are: the leafy parts of edible plants. Each one is unique and individual with its own texture and flavor. Some are bitter, a taste some folks don't like. Others, though, are sweet, some are sour, and still others have an amazing and startling bite! Some are spicy and some are not. Because of the incredible variety, I encourage you to try them all, and then choose those that are your favorites for your daily eating. Remember, shake it up and eat a variety. Each of these types are not only unique in flavor, but also in nutrient makeup. Your highest and best health will come from rotating through as many as possible.

This is by no means a complete list, but leafy greens include:

Arugula	Dandelion Greens	Purslane
Basil	Fennel	Radicchio
Beet Greens	Kale	Rapini
Bok Choy	Lettuce	Spinach
Cabbage	Mustard Greens	Swiss Chard
Celery Leaves	Napa Cabbage	Turnip Greens
Collard Greens	Plantain	Watercress

Most of these can be found in markets with well-stocked produce sections. Purslane is considered a weed by the uninformed, and is likely to be found within 100 feet of your front door during the warmer seasons. Purslane, along with other leafy greens not stocked in your local market, can typically be ordered if you ask the produce manager.

I also recommend visiting ethnic markets and local farmer's markets if they are to be found in your area. Asian, Indian, and Mexican markets abound with cool new greens to try, and small farmers love to grow and share new things. Farmer's markets are also the best way to acquire and consume fruits and vegetables in their proper season. There is no tastier or more nutritious way to eat produce. Read up on them and you may be surprised at the thrilling dishes you can create.

Serving size: A serving of leafy greens is 3 lightly packed cups if raw, or 1 cup if cooked. The exceptions are cabbages, which are 1½ cups if raw, 1 cup if cooked. The difference between raw and cooked is due to the tendency of greens to break down and wilt during cooking.

GROUP 2 - VEGETABLES

This group is separated from leafy greens because leafy greens, by and large, offer the greatest nutrient density of all vegetables and are therefore more important to daily eating. There are many other great veggies to be added, though, but be cautious: some are better suited to the carb group I will share in a bit.

Important veggies include, but again are by no means limited to:

Artichokes	Brussels Sprouts	Kohlrabi
Asparagus	Cauliflower	Leeks
Bean Sprouts	Celery	Mushrooms
Bell Peppers	Eggplants	Okra
Broccoli	Garlic	Onions
Broccolini	Green Beans	Zucchini

As with leafy greens, it is fun to frequent ethnic markets and farmer's markets to discover new tasty treats in the veggie group.

Serving size: A serving of veggies (other than leafy greens) is 1 cup raw.

GROUP 3 - PROTEINS

This group is composed primarily, though not entirely, of meats. Beef, pork, lamb, fowl, and seafood of all types are packed with protein. If it once walked, flew, swam, or slithered along, it is made of protein.

If you have chosen a vegetarian or vegan lifestyle, you need to be aware that there are a number of nutrients that are harder to come by without animal products. Don't get me wrong, there are benefits to a plant-based diet; however, you have to be aware of those harder-to-come-by nutrients and ensure you get enough of them. And by "get them," I mean from food, not from supplements. These nutrients include vitamins B12 and D3, heme-iron, zinc, and omega-3 fatty acids. If you intend to pursue a vegetarian or vegan lifestyle, I encourage you to do additional reading to ensure you consume enough proteins and the more difficult nutrients in adequate supply for your metabolism. I provide some options here, but there are many more that are not covered in the context of this book.

Stay away from ultra-processed meats like lunch meats and most breakfast sausages. Be very careful which type of bacon you choose. Again, read ingredient labels. You should know the source of ground meats; it is best to have your butcher grind your meats while you watch. Also avoid meats from fast food sources. You want meats, not chemicals or meat-like substances.

You have likely also heard about CAFO (concentrated animal feeding operation) factories. These are the source for most beef, pork, and fowl found in your supermarket. These meats can be polluted in all sorts of ways and, because of that fact, are pumped full of huge concentrations of antibiotics. Although it can be a bit more expensive in some places, it is best to look for grass-fed beef, free-range fowl, and wild-caught seafood. If you can find locally-raised meats, that's even better. Local farmer's markets can be great sources for high quality meats. Again, do the best you can do based on what is available where you live, and at a price you can afford.

Protein can be found in plants, yes, in varying degrees. All grains are protein sources. Quinoa, in fact, is a perfect protein, meaning it contains all nine amino acids that your metabolism cannot make for itself. Other high protein grains include oats, spelt, kamut, amaranth, bulgur, and many more.

Remember when using grains as protein, they must also be counted against your carbs from Group 4.

Many green plants have protein as well! One of the best protein sources anywhere is that same little-known leafy green mentioned above, purslane: a weed to most folks, growing out of the cracks in concrete or wherever else it can get a foothold. Most markets can order it for you. Other green vegetable protein sources include broccoli, spinach, Brussels sprouts, and collard greens. Additional plant proteins include tofu, seitan, and tempeh.

And don't forget seafood. Freshwater and ocean fish, crabs, lobster and shrimps are delicious protein sources.

You may be aware of other amazing protein sources. Some may be unique to your culture or your geographic location. I would love to hear about them!

Serving size: A serving of meat protein is 4 to 6 ounces before cooking. A serving of grain-based protein is ¾ cup, cooked. Green plant proteins can be eaten in as large a quantity as you wish, though you should have at least 1 cup cooked.

GROUP 4 - CARBS

Carbs are essential for optimal health, as we discussed in earlier chapters; don't let any fad blogger tell you differently.

There is a lot of chatter in the media and blogs about *simple* carbs and *complex* carbs. That is misdirection at its finest. There are quite literally hundreds of levels of complexity in carbohydrate molecules. To cast them into two broad classes, and then to proclaim one class better than the other, is just silly. Instead, we ought to think of carbs in these two categories: processed carbs and unprocessed carbs. Avoid processed carbs. Eat unprocessed carbs. Simple.

Healthy carbs include all fruits, including fruits we think of as vegetables such as tomatoes; pumpkin and winter squashes; avocados; and the like.

Carbs also include starches: root vegetables like potatoes, carrots, beets, and yams; and all kinds of beans, lentils, and peas.

Other carbs that you may not think of as such are dairy products, including milk, cream, cheese, and yogurt. Peanut butter belongs in the carb group, along with peanuts, all tree nuts, and legumes.

Corn is a carb. I give corn its own line because I have heard people call it a fruit, a vegetable, and a grain. It is, curiously, a grain if harvested when the seeds are dry, but a vegetable if harvested when the seeds are plump. How's that for confusing? It is a carb, regardless when it is harvested, however.

And, of course, grains are carbs. Remember though, that some grains are also great sources of vegetarian protein. If used as protein, they must be counted as a carb serving as well.

Serving size: With carbs, serving size gets a bit trickier. The following are general guidelines.

- *Dairy - 1 cup whole milk, 1/3 cup ice cream or yogurt, cheese about the size of 4 dice or 1 slice, 1 tablespoon butter*
- *Nuts - about 7 nuts or two level tablespoons nut butter (not the standard heaping spoon we wish it were)*
- *Grains - ¾ cup cooked*
- *Fruits - equivalent to roughly the size of a medium orange or apple, or ½ cup berries*
- *Corn, beans, or lentils - ¾ cup*
- *Starchy root vegetables - 1 cup*

Balancing the Four Groups in Meals

Now that we have established the four groups, let's look at meal planning. This looks incredibly simple, and it is. Don't allow the simplicity to dissuade you, though; this is what eating looked like for thousands of years before the industrial revolution brought factory processing into the picture.

Portion sizes are not as important as you may think. Balance is the key. If you eat foods in the correct proportions to one another, and stop eating when your hunger has been sated, the actual portion size is much less important. Use the portion sizes listed as guides—starting points. After talking about each meal, I will show you how to adjust for your personal level of hunger. No one should ever go hungry just because of an eating plan, after all.

Breakfast

It is best if breakfast is kept on the lighter side. A small portion of a carb is okay for breakfast, although most people will be more satisfied if this meal is primarily protein. A great breakfast is an egg and a small amount of another protein: a piece of bacon, for example, or one-third cup (cooked) oats or quinoa. If you have a very active job with lots of heavy lifting or constant motion, you may wish to add a carb to your breakfast, preferably a fruit, or you may favor grain-based proteins. If you have grains without eggs, have a ¾ cup, cooked, serving.

Lunch

Lunch should include:

- 1 serving from Group 1 (leafy greens)
- ½ to 1 serving from Group 2 (veggies).

160

- 1 serving from Group 3 (proteins).
- 1 serving from Group 4 (carbs).

Remember, if a grain is used as a protein, it also counts as your carb for that meal.

Dinner

Dinner follows the same balance as lunch.

Hunger

Hunger kills any healthy eating plan. When you become excessively hungry, you will most likely head straight to carbs, completely upending your carb balance. Managing hunger is easy, though. Get all of your water, leafy greens, and veggies first. Those are your highest priority. After that, just keep your proteins and carbs in balance. For example, if you are hungry after a meal, add 3 more ounces of protein and half of a fruit. That is one-half of a serving of each, which keeps the two in balance. Conversely, if you are becoming over-full, decrease your protein and carb in the same balance. Easy, right?

Snacks

Don't snack. My mom always told us kids that eating between meals spoils dinner, and she was right. There are a lot of pop diets out there telling you to eat several smaller meals throughout the day, or to allow protein snacks. There is no quantifiable science behind that advice, and it actually makes healthy, balanced eating much more difficult. This is because of a little gremlin, or rather a hormone called *ghrelin*.

Ghrelin is commonly called the *hunger hormone*. There are two specific events that trigger this hormone, making you feel hunger.

The first trigger is a deprivation of nutrients. Most folks think you feel hunger when your stomach is empty, but that is not how it really works. You may have had the experience of filling your stomach, maybe eating too much even, and still feeling hungry. Your body is not looking for additional volume of food; it is looking for adequate nutrition. If you provide that nutrition, you feel satisfied. If you provide only filler food, devoid of those nutrients, you still feel hunger.

The second trigger of ghrelin is less known, but far craftier. Your body has an internal timekeeper we call your *circadian rhythm*, or "body clock," which is programmed by your habits. If you have a habit of eating near a certain time most days, your body will automatically produce ghrelin at that time, making sure you don't forget to eat. Now, if it is your habit to eat several times a day (and that includes snacking, coffees full of cream or spices, and so forth) you can see what happens, right? You are constantly producing ghrelin and, therefore, always hungry.

That is why, even if your snack food choices are the healthiest foods on earth, the very *habit* of snacking is one of the unhealthiest things you can do. It is important to stick to your normal three meals a day, as a rule, and to get all of your food at those meals.

If you have been in the habit of snacking through the day, it is important to change that habit. For a couple of weeks, because of ghrelin, breaking the snacking habit can be pretty hard. Couple that with a little stress and the way we have been manipulated to look for so-called comfort foods and BAM! However, after eliminating snacking for about two weeks, your circadian rhythms will begin to reprogram themselves and ghrelin will stop bothering you at those times. And once free of ghrelin, it becomes easier to argue with our stress and avoid emotional eating as well. Hard though it may be at first, you will be happier and feel better after eliminating the snacking habit.

Alcohol

Not surprisingly, I get this question a lot: "Can I still drink wine or other alcohol?" Yes, you can. Alcohol is a carb, and should be treated as such. On the days you drink alcohol, reduce your carbs at meal times; your alcohol will be your carb for that day. Obviously, though, alcohol is not the highest quality carb, so you do not want to drink every day because you will never get enough of the healthier carbs. But occasionally it is just fine.

What about holidays and other special meals or nights out?

Listen, occasional indulgence has been a part of the human experience since the beginning of humans. Seasonal festivals, including excess food and drink, are found all throughout recorded history, and archeological evidence suggests their occurrence reaches back even further. They are part of the quality of life and we should enjoy them.

Occasionally.

There is a cool phenomenon in your body that causes it to ignore anomalous eating. In other words, if you eat in a healthy manner every day and only occasionally indulge, your metabolism will pass off the added junk and imbalance and just ignore it.

The problem in our society today is that "special" occasions are not so special anymore; they happen all the time. In some circles, there is a party every week. Worse, we are collectively conditioned to eat garbage at every event we attend, even markedly UN-special events like driving home or trips to the mall. If imbalanced eating becomes habit instead of anomaly, your metabolism begins to stress and plan for the crisis that is malnutrition.

Keep special occasions *occasional*, and you will have no problem.

Chapter Nineteen
Your Results—What to Expect

What can you expect if you follow Shiwu Zen? You can expect results equal to the degree to which you follow the plan. With consistency you will see marked improvement over time in your blood pressure, cholesterol, blood sugar, and triglycerides. Many Nutri-90 clients also report improvements with sleep apnea, pre-diabetes, and other nutrition related disorders. And yes, you can see sustainable weight loss, even dramatic weight loss.

There are three ways folks tend to sabotage themselves, though. Let's talk about them so that you can avoid the pitfalls and see permanent success for yourself in reaching your goals.

The three biggest mistakes clients make are the three "little things" they believe won't matter: not getting enough water, not eating enough leafy greens, and sneaking in processed foods laden with chemical additives. Those things do matter. Your results could slow or even stop because of those deviations.

There is one more mistake I see from time to time. I have witnessed clients who experience amazing results and then… just stop. That often happens because of associations tied to the word "diet." Clinically, diet means what you eat, whatever that may be. When you hear, "that guy should improve his diet," it means that guy should eat differently. However, words do mean things, and in the popular context *diet* has come to mean something special to do for a short time in order to lose weight or meet a health goal, after which a person turns the diet off and goes back to "normal eating." After amazing results, someone may "turn off the diet" and return to the same "normal" eating habits that led to obesity and loss of vitality in the first place. If you do that, if you stop even after seeing and feeling amazing results, there is only one eventuality you can reasonably expect: returning to poor eating will quickly transport you right back to where you began, and maybe even further out of sync than you were when you started.

The thing to understand is that Shiwu Zen is exactly what normal eating meant for thousands of years. The garbage that folks crave today did not even exist a century ago, and can therefore hardly be called normal. To your body, modern "normal food" is toxic poison. It is sickening the population. Just look around yourself for proof of that. Shiwu Zen *is* normal eating.

If you understand that and accept Shiwu Zen as your new normal, you can expect your lab results to improve at your next physician checkup, you can expect more energy, and you can expect weight loss. How much? That depends on you and your biological makeup, but you ought to see steady results.

You may have friends or family who have joined Nutri-90 and have experienced spectacular weight loss, health and wellness improvements, and increased mobility and vitality. Nutri-90 creates specific coaching plans for our clients which address their unique needs and challenges. Because all client plans are personalized to the unique individual, results tend to be faster and more impressive. Check our website for information if you are ready to take the next step toward your personal vitality, weight loss, and wellness. You can learn more and start your own journey to metabolic optimization at nutri-90.com

Chapter Twenty
Who Knew Real Food Tasted So Good?

No, this is not a recipe book, but I do want you to experience how delicious real, honest food can be. Food preparation is almost a lost art, but it isn't hard. Think about it; 60 years ago, nearly every family cooked every meal. Wow, right?

But they had more time to cook, and food was less expensive, and all that... isn't that true? No, it isn't. With these recipes, you can feed your family for a lower cost than that of most fast food, and prep time can be less than the average lunch hour wait at your local burger joint. All it takes is a new mindset and a little forethought.

Be forewarned, I am not a master chef. But these recipes are not meant for people with all the time in the world and a kitchen to die for. They are meant for real, normal people with responsibilities and a life, people like you and me. And you know what? They are *still* delicious enough that you will want to serve them to friends!

Note that leafy greens are prepared three different ways in these recipes: baked, steamed, and in soup. Try all three and see which is your favorite!

Before we get into the recipes, here are a few general notes that will make your experience with these recipes even better.

General Recipe Notes

Tiny Kitchen: These recipes reference Tiny Kitchen seasoning blends. Most seasonings at the supermarkets are designed for recipes utilizing processed foods, and are therefore not as good when cooking with real, fresh foods. Tiny Kitchen seasonings are extraordinarily crafted to deliciously marry the flavors of non-processed vegetables, fruits, and meats. Tiny Kitchen seasonings are found at   shop.nutri-90.com

If you choose to substitute other seasonings in place of Tiny Kitchen seasonings, I would recommend the following:

Broccoli Chip: substitute with 2 parts celery salt and 1 part dill weed.

Seafood Splash: substitute with Old Bay Seasoning.

Baja Blend: substitute with taco seasoning. Baja Blend is unique, though, and I would highly recommend getting some and trying it out.

Celery Salt: substitute with celery salt.

Great China: substitute with 3 parts Chinese five spice and 1 part ground black pepper

Clean Seasonings and Sauces: Popular seasonings and sauces in stores very often contain fillers, anti-caking agents, excessive sugars and salt, preservatives, and artificial colors and flavors. Always read labels carefully and choose clean seasonings and sauces, ones which are free of such toxic substances.

Stevia: There is some controversy surrounding stevia-based sweeteners. As always, read ingredient labels carefully and make yourself knowledgeable about what those ingredients are. Not all stevia-based sweeteners are the same, and I have learned that formulations can vary from region to region even within the same brand. I leave the choice to you, but always use caution in making selections.

Presentation: Food tastes better when it looks appealing; it is just a fact about the relationship between what you see and what you taste. Therefore, when you work to prepare a tasty dish for your family or friends, also take the time to plate it, that is to say present it, in an exciting, tempting way.

I watch local discount stores and thrift stores for interesting plates, glasses, and flatware I can use at dinnertime. Antiques are also appealing. I have found with my family that serving everyone on a different style of plate can be really fun, adding another layer to the enjoyment of mealtime and the food prepared.

There was a time when an important part of family time was spent at the dinner table. In many countries that still holds true. I think you will find that your family will enjoy the same connections, and your family becomes stronger when meals are both nourishing and playful. Give it a try!

Now turn the page for some real deliciousness.

Pepper Pot Soup

A traditional East Indies dish from centuries past, I first tasted this hearty and delicious soup when visiting Philadelphia. The story has it that certain colonial settlers, who may also have founded a fledgling nation along the way, visited the East Indies and brought this recipe back with them. True or not, we are the winners when we prepare and indulge in this spicy recipe, which is sure to warm our hearts and souls on the chilliest of evenings.

Ingredients:

- 1½ pounds salt-cured pork loin, diced (see chef's note)
- 1 medium white onion, chopped
- 4 cloves garlic, minced
- ¼ habanero pepper, seeded and minced (see chef's note)
- 1 cup scallions, chopped
- 1 pound taro root, peeled and diced (see chef's note)
- 1 gallon chicken stock (see chef's note)
- 2 bay leaves
- 1 teaspoon fresh thyme, chopped
- 1 tablespoon freshly ground allspice (see chef's note)
- 1 tablespoon freshly ground black pepper, plus more (see chef's note)
- 1 pound callaloo or collard greens, rinsed and chopped (see chef's note)

Method:

In a large, well-seasoned cast-iron skillet or carbon steel wok, sauté the pork over high heat for 10 minutes or until browned. Keep meat moving with spatula to avoid sticking. Add the onions, garlic, and habanero pepper and sauté for 3 to 5 minutes, until the onion starts to become translucent. Add the scallions and sauté for 3 minutes. Add the taro root and sauté for 3 to 5 minutes more, until translucent.

Transfer contents of skillet to a large stock pot and add 4 cups of chicken stock. Place over high heat.

Add 1 cup chicken stock to the still-hot skillet and deglaze. Pour this liquid into stock pot. Add bay leaves, thyme, allspice, and pepper. Add remaining chicken stock and bring to boil over high heat. Reduce heat to medium and cook for about 30 minutes, until the meat and taro root are tender.

Stir in the greens (callaloo or collard greens) and simmer on low heat for about 5 minutes, until greens are wilted. Serve hot.

Makes 8 to 12 servings.

Chef's Notes:

1 - You may use fresh pork if you wish, but salt pork, which was the method of meat preservation in colonial days, preserves the original subtleties of the dish. To salt-cure pork at home, start at least five days before preparing this dish. Rub whole pork loin generously on all sides with coarse-ground sea salt. Make sure the entire loin is encrusted with the salt. Seal tightly in a large sealable bag. Place in the refrigerator and turn daily for at least three days; I find five days gives the best result. Remove the loin from bag and rinse vigorously before slicing or dicing.
2 - Habanero pepper is very, VERY hot. I strongly urge wearing disposable kitchen gloves when handling this pepper, then washing your hands well before touching your face. If spicy-hot dishes are not for you, simply leave this pepper out of the recipe.
3 - Taro root can sometimes be hard to find. If unavailable, turmeric root works, adding its own unique flourish.
4 - Allspice loses some of its amazing olfactory bliss and taste very quickly after it is ground. For best results, buy whole allspice berries and either grind in a coffee grinder or crush with a mortar and pestle just before use.
5 - During cooking, black pepper has a volatile element that cooks away. This leaves a very pleasant flavor behind, but for best results it is good to add an additional ¼ teaspoon of ground black pepper just before serving.
6 – Callaloo in this recipe refers to the leafy green tops of the taro root. In some communities this is easy to find, but in many locales you will need to use collard greens instead. The flavor integrity of the dish remains with either of these two greens.

Jumbo Shrimp & Broccoli Stir Fry

There are two pervasive myths that have entwined themselves throughout the world of healthy eating. The first proclaims that healthy cooking takes too long and is hard to learn. The second holds that healthy foods cost too much. This Tiny Kitchen recipe shoots down both of those fables. Feed a family of three and make your friends think you are a master chef in just 15 minutes and with only $10.

Ingredients:
- 1 pound jumbo shrimp (deveined, skins on or off, your choice)
- 4 cups fresh broccoli
- 4 cloves garlic, minced
- ½-inch piece ginger root, minced
- 1 teaspoon Tiny Kitchen Seafood Splash Seasoning
- A few shakes of Tiny Kitchen Celery Salt
- White balsamic vinegar (about ½ cup)
- Lemon juice (about ¼ cup in spritzer or food grade spray bottle)
- 2 teaspoons stevia-based sweetener or to taste
- 2 bunches mustard greens

Method:

In saucepan over medium heat, add white balsamic vinegar, garlic, ginger, 5 or 6 spritzes of lemon juice, and Tiny Kitchen Seafood Splash Seasoning. Stir together and allow mixture to just barely come to a boil. Reduce heat to low, stir well, and simmer on rear burner.

You are making a reduction sauce. Begin preparing shrimp and broccoli while keeping an eye on the sauce. When it reaches a slightly thicker consistency which just starts clinging to your spoon, add stevia-based sweetener and stir well; allow to simmer two minutes more, then turn heat off.

Cook broccoli in microwave on high for 2 minutes and 30 seconds. You can add ¼ cup water to the dish if desired, or microwave dry; both will yield favorable results. Be sure to use a microwave-safe dish.

Place a well-seasoned wok over medium-high heat, then add shrimp once hot. Keep shrimp moving and cook only until bright pink on all sides; do not fully cook yet. Remove shrimp from pan and set aside.

Reduce heat to medium and add pre-cooked broccoli along with a few shakes of Tiny Kitchen Celery Salt. Broccoli should still be crunchy, even though it has been heated in the microwave. Toss broccoli in wok for 1 minute, then add shrimp back in. Keep moving in wok until shrimp are cooked through, about 5 minutes. Remove from heat.

Remove the thick stems of the mustard greens and discard. Chop or tear the leaves into course pieces and cook in microwave on high for 1 minute and 30 seconds.

Your reduction sauce should be finishing up about this same time. If sauce has not begun to get a little syrupy yet, raise heat until it just starts to bubble and watch it carefully until it begins to thicken, then reduce heat and add stevia-based sweetener; finish as directed above.

Place a bed of mustard greens on a plate and add about 1½ cups of shrimp and broccoli on top of it. Spoon Ginger Garlic Sauce over cooked shrimp and broccoli and serve immediately!

Makes four servings.

Crock Pot Adobo

Crock pot cooking is da BOMB for great taste with minimal prep time, and this Crock Pot Adobo really brings it home. Adobo is a sweet, salty cooking method that makes even tough meats soft, juicy, and delicious; it's a favorite in Mexico and Spain but really made special in the Philippines, where every region adds its own twist. Give this a try; I bet it immediately becomes one of your family favorites. (And wait until you see how simple it is!)

Ingredients:

- 1 medium pork loin, cut into ¾-inch cubes
- 1½ cups chicken broth
- ½ cup soy sauce
- ¼ cup cane vinegar (available from most Asian markets)
- 4 cloves garlic
- 1 teaspoon whole black peppercorns
- 1 teaspoon stevia-based sweetener
- 2-3 bay leaves
- 1 teaspoon sea salt
- 6 cups spinach, washed and drained

Method:

On the night before you will serve this dish:

Mix soy sauce, garlic, peppercorns, stevia-based sweetener, bay leaves, and salt well. Add pork and put into a large sealable storage bag. Shake well, until meat is completely coated. Squeeze excess air out of bag, reseal, and let stand in the refrigerator overnight.

On the morning of the day you will serve this dish:

Empty all contents of the marinade bag into a crock pot. Add the chicken broth. Cover crock pot and cook on low for 8 hours.

One half-hour before dinner time:

> Add the cane vinegar and salt; stir and cook on high for the final half-hour of your cooking time.
>
> While cooking is completing, prepare your vegetable for the evening. I recommend steamed spinach with Tiny Kitchen Broccoli Chip Seasoning; the flavors marry marvelously with adobo. Cook the spinach in microwave on high for 1 minute. Place about a cup of the cooked spinach on each plate under a 1-cup serving of adobo. Remember, it takes about three cups of raw spinach to make 1 cup cooked.

Serve hot.

The leftovers of this dish are also great-tasting cold for lunches, or reheated for other meals.

Makes four to six servings.

Baked Kale and Pork

You don't have to be a culinary expert or a world class chef to prepare this amazing recipe, but your friends will think you are. This is so easy that my personal assistant's teenage daughter made it for us; it took her 25 minutes in the kitchen, and when she brought it to the table, the scent was mouthwatering. And the taste... well... wow.

Ingredients:

- 2 pork loin chops, thinly sliced
- 2 bunches kale
- 2 Granny Smith apples, seeds removed and cut into wedges
- White balsamic vinegar (about ¾ cup)
- Lemon juice (about ¼ cup in spritzer or food-grade spray bottle)
- Tiny Kitchen Baja Blend Seasoning
- Tiny Kitchen Broccoli Chip Seasoning
- 1 teaspoon cinnamon
- 1 teaspoon stevia-based sweetener

Method:

Preheat oven to 400° F.

Heat skillet (preferably cast iron) over medium heat.

Remove thick stems from kale and tear leaves into largish chunks. Arrange leaves in bottom section of broiler pan or high-sided cookie sheet. Set aside.

Sprinkle pork liberally on both sides with Tiny Kitchen Baja Blend Seasoning. Place in un-oiled skillet and begin to sear. When bottom begins to brown, add about ¼ cup white balsamic vinegar to pan. Flip pork and sear other side. Do not cook through; just brown each side, then remove from skillet and set aside.

With skillet still over medium heat, deglaze pan by adding ½ cup white balsamic vinegar and lightly scraping meat and seasoning residue from bottom of pan with the edge of a fork or a spatula as the vinegar begins to bubble. Add cinnamon and stir, and then add apple wedges, skin side up. Stir a bit, turning apples from side to side occasionally, until liquid is reduced by half. Reduce heat to simmer; add stevia-based sweetener and allow liquid to reduce by half again, stirring and turning apple wedges occasionally. When sauce is reduced, remove skillet from heat and set aside.

While sauce is reducing, spritz kale evenly with lemon juice and sprinkle with Tiny Kitchen Broccoli Chip Seasoning to taste. Put pork on top of kale and place on center rack of oven. Set timer for 15 minutes.

When timer sounds, check pork by making a cut in the center of the thickest piece. Pork is done if juices are clear with no pink.

Plate kale with pork loin chop on top and apple wedges to the side, then spoon a bit of the sauce over the pork and apples. Presentation affects the taste of food psychologically, so take a few moments to make it pretty and appealing.

Makes 2 servings.

Poached White Fish

If you have ever baked or fried white fish, fish such as cod, swai, tilapia, and so on, you know how easy it dries out and becomes tasteless, with the consistency of cardboard. In fact, it can be almost impossible to avoid! But fret not; there is an easy method for cooking white fish that yields a juicy, delicious dish every time: poaching. The technique is easy to master by following these simple directions, which will yield amazing food for you, your family, and your guests.

Ingredients:

- Ling cod fillet, cut into two pieces (any white fish works)
- 4 cups baby kale and chard mix
- 2 navel oranges, wedged
- ½ cup chicken broth (prepared earlier), divided
- 3 teaspoons Tiny Kitchen Great China Seasoning, divided
- 1½ teaspoons Tiny Kitchen Broccoli Chip Seasoning or to taste
- 2 pieces star anise (optional)

Method:

Prep kale and chard mix by pulsing in a food processor until chopped into small pieces. Stop before it starts to liquefy. Add Tiny Kitchen Broccoli Chip Seasoning to taste, pulse two or three times more, and set aside.

Place a high sided skillet with a close fitting lid over medium heat and add ¼ cup chicken broth.

Sprinkle Tiny Kitchen Great China Seasoning on both sides of fish fillets, using about 1½ teaspoons total.

As broth heats, add orange wedges in an even layer; do not allow to stack on top of one another. Add 1½ teaspoon Tiny Kitchen Great China Seasoning to broth and stir. Adjust layer of oranges. When broth is beginning to bubble, add remaining ¼ cup chicken broth and star anise, and arrange fish fillets over oranges. Rest fish entirely on orange wedges; do not allow to touch bottom of pan. Cover with lid and poach (steam) over medium heat for 8 to 10 minutes, depending on thickness of fish.

When fish is done cooking (opaque all the way through), lay a bed of the prepared greens on the bottom of your plate and place the fish carefully on top. Set plate aside for fish to rest.

While fish is resting, turn up heat under skillet to medium high and reduce the liquid without lid until liquid begins to thicken just a bit. Spoon glaze over fish (don't use too much) and serve. Delicious and beautiful!

Makes two servings.

Pollo Asado de Baja

What is sweet, tangy, spicy, and meaty, all in the same dish? Well, Pollo Asado de Baja, of course! This one-dish recipe is so delicious you will never believe you can lose weight while eating it, but you will. This meal is well-balanced nutritionally and stimulates the body to release stored body fat.

Ingredients:

- 3 chicken breasts, cut into quarters
- 1 medium onion, chopped into eights and sections separated
- 6-8 cloves garlic
- 4 tomatoes, quartered
- 1 bunch Asparagus
- ⅛ cup white balsamic vinegar, plus more
- 2-3 teaspoons Tiny Kitchen Baja Blend Seasoning
- Tiny Kitchen Broccoli Chip Seasoning
- 3 bunches dandelion greens (or mustard greens)

Method:

Prep garlic by cutting a smiley face-shape into the side of each clove.

Place chicken pieces into large sealable storage bag, add Tiny Kitchen Baja Seasoning, seal bag, and shake until seasoning covers chicken thoroughly.

Set prep aside and heat a large high-sided skillet with a close-fitting lid over medium heat. Sauté onion and garlic until just starting to become translucent and the delicious scent is released. Because we are not using oil, keep ingredients in motion in skillet at all times to prevent sticking. Add white balsamic vinegar and toss well.

When vinegar just starts to bubble, level the onions and garlic into a single layer in bottom of pan. Arrange tomatoes in pan evenly. Arrange chicken in the same manner as the tomatoes. Chicken and tomatoes should form a single layer in the pan when this is complete. Add enough white balsamic vinegar to cover garlic and onion layer, but not enough to get much into the chicken.

Bring the vinegar barely to a boil; place tight fitting lid onto skillet, allow pan to fill with steam, and then reduce heat to simmer. Allow to simmer like this for 40 minutes.

About 5 minutes before Pollo Asado is ready, remove the white woody section from the asparagus and discard. Cut remaining asparagus into pieces about 1" long. Place these pieces in a microwave safe bowl, sprinkle liberally with Tiny Kitchen Broccoli Chip Seasoning, then steam on high in microwave for 2 minutes and 30 seconds.

Serve in a medium sized bowl, Pollo Asado on one side spooned over fresh dandelion greens, and asparagus on the other. Mmmm-mmmm, good eats!

Makes 3 servings.

The Best Damned Wings

All right, all right. You have been asking. Begging even. "What can I eat on Game Day? How can I party of the fourth of July? Give me something I can eat that just screams 'fun!'" you say. Well, honestly I can't blame you.

So let's talk wings. What food screams "TAILGATE" louder than scorching hot wings? The crispier the better, and did I mention HOT?! Now I normally save this recipe for Super Bowl Weekend, but I know you want something a little different sometimes, just to cut loose.

The secret to a super crisp, non-floured, non-fried wing recipe is a simple technique called parboiling. More on that in a minute, okay? First, here is what you will need.

Ingredients:

- 2 pounds chicken wings, thawed
- 5 tablespoons Tabasco, or other clean hot sauce*
- 3 cloves garlic, minced
- Cayenne pepper
- Salt

*a clean hot sauce contains only peppers, vinegar, and maybe salt

So far, pretty easy, right? You will also need a gallon-sized sealable bag, a cookie sheet lined with aluminum foil, a largish soup pot for boiling water, a sauce pan, and some paper towels.

Method:

Fill soup pot half-full of water. Add enough salt to make it taste a bit over-salty, like sea water. Place on burner over high heat and bring to boil.

Preheat oven to 450° F.

While everything is heating up, take a moment to rinse your thawed wings under cold water.

When water is boiling hard, slowly and carefully place wings into your soup pot. Depending on the size of your pot, you may have to parboil your wings one pound at a time. Parboiling will remove much of the fat, and removing the thicker areas of fat will allow the wings to crisp up nicely later. It will also cause the water to foam, so watch your pot carefully and reduce heat to avoid foam-over if necessary. Boil wings for 7 minutes.

Remove wings from boiling water to a cooling rack, if you have one, or onto a generous mat of paper towels. Allow to dry for 4 or 5 minutes, then roll them over and allow to dry 2 minutes more.

While chicken is drying, mix hot sauce, garlic, ½ teaspoon cayenne pepper (or to taste), and ½ teaspoon salt in a sauce pan and place over medium heat, until hot and well-blended.

Place dried wings on cookie sheet lined with foil. Sprinkle all sides with a little salt and a fairly liberal sprinkling of cayenne pepper.

Place wings in hot oven for 25 to 30 minutes, depending on the size of your wings. Flip them all and bake another 5 minutes. Baked wings should be a crispy, golden brown. Allow to cool 5 minutes or so.

Place wings in sealable bag. Using a spatula, scrape all of the sauce from the sauce pan into the bag. Fill with air and seal. Now roll the bag over and over until all wings are evenly coated with the sauce.

That's it! Serve hot or cooled, your choice.

Bon appétit, folks! And by the way, there is no reason at all to believe weight loss food has to be boring, tasteless, or bland.

A serving is about 5 to 7 wings.

Endnotes

---

[1] Rohit Malik, Catch Me If You Can: Big Food Using Big Tobacco's Playbook? Applying the Lessons Learned from Big Tobacco to Attack the Obesity Epidemic (2010).

[2] "U.S. Weight Loss Market Worth $60.9 Billion," last modified May 09, 2011, http://www.prweb.com/releases/2011/5/prweb8393658.htm. May 2011

[3] Christopher JL Murray, et al., "UK health performance: findings of the Global Burden of Disease Study 2010," The Lancet 381, no. 9871 (March 2013): 997-1020, doi: http://dx.doi.org/10.1016/S0140-6736(13)60355-4

[4] See note 3 above.

[5] NIH Technology Assessment Conference Panel, "Methods for Voluntary Weight Loss and Control," Ann Intern Med. (1992):116:942-949. doi:10.7326/0003-4819-116-11-942

[6] "Multivitamins are, at best, a waste of money, Johns Hopkins doctors say," Hub Staff Report, December 17, 2013, http://hub.jhu.edu/2013/12/17/vitamins-might-be-harmful

[7] Farin Kamingar and Ashkan Emadi, "Vitamin and Mineral Supplements: Do We Really Need Them?" International Journal of Preventative Medicine 3.3 (2012): 221-226.

[8] Konrad Heindorff, et al., "Genetic toxicology of ethylenediaminetetraacetic acid (EDTA)," Mutation Research/Reviews in Genetic Toxicology 115, no. 2 (June 1983): 149-173, doi:10.1016/0165-1110(83)90001-5, http://www.sciencedirect.com/science/article/pii/0165111083900015

[9] "The Obesity Paradox: Overfed but Undernourished," Kristin Wartman, The Huffington Post Online, June 28, 2012, http://www.americarecordnews.win/kristin-wartman/the-obesity-paradox_b_1632862.html

[10] Belldon Colme and Nutri-90 "Give Back" to the community through monetary contributions and by conducting nutrition workshops in elementary schools.

[11] "Role of proteins in the body," University of Waikato, June 10, 2011, http://sciencelearn.org.nz/Contexts/Uniquely-Me/Science-Ideas-and-Concepts/Role-of-proteins-in-the-body

[12] "So Many Proteins, So Much Promise," Megan Fellman, October 31, 2011, http://www.northwestern.edu/newscenter/stories/2011/10/proteomics-kelleher.html

[13] "The Dangers of Treating Obesity as a Disability," The Chicago Tribune Online, December 29, 2014, http://www.chicagotribune.com/news/opinion/editorials/ct-obesity-ada-disability-eu-court-of-justice-edit-1229-jm-20141226-story.html

[14] James L. Hargrove, "History of the Calorie in Nutrition," The Journal of Nutrition, vol. 136 no. 12, (2006): 2957-2961

[15] "Caloric," The Free Dictionary, http://www.thefreedictionary.com/caloric

[16] James L. Hargrove, "Does the history of food energy units suggest a solution to 'Calorie confusion'?" Nutrition Journal 6 (2007): 44, doi:10.1186/1475-2891-6-44

[17] Annabel L. Merrill and Bernice K. Watt, Energy Value of Foods... Basis and Derivation: Agriculture Handbook No. 74 (Washington, D.C.: U.S. Government Printing Office, 1973).

[18] "Killing Off the Calorie," *Big Picture: Food and Diet*, Summer 2011, http://bigpictureeducation.com/killing-calorie

[19] Chin Jou, "Counting Calories," *Chemical Heritage*, Spring 2011, http://www.chemheritage.org/discover/media/magazine/articles/29-1-counting-calories.aspx

[20] James A. Madura and John K. DiBaise, "Quick fix or long-term cure? Pros and cons of bariatric surgery," *F1000 Medicine Reports* 4 (2012): 19, doi: 10.3410/M4-19

[21] "Laser liposuction—weight loss tool or scam?," Caroline Novas, 2011, http://center4research.org/i-saw-it-on-the-internet/laser-liposuction-weight-loss-tool-or-scam/

[22] "The Miracle Weight Loss that Isn't," Sabrina Rubin Erdely, last modified August 18, 2008, http://www.nbcnews.com/id/26076054/ns/health-diet_and_nutrition/t/miracle-weight-loss-isnt/

[23] "Columbia and the Problem of Dr. Oz," Michael Specter, *The New Yorker*, April 23, 2015, http://www.newyorker.com/news/daily-comment/columbia-and-the-problem-of-dr-oz

[24] "General Mills, Inc. 5/5/09," Food and Drug Administration, last modified June 18, 2009, http://www.fda.gov/ICECI/EnforcementActions/WarningLetters/ucm162943.htm

[25] "The Hidden Costs of Hamburgers," Ellen Rolfes, *PBS NewsHour*, August 2, 2012, http://www.pbs.org/newshour/rundown/the-hidden-costs-of-hamburgers/

[26] Kelly M. Adams, Martin Kohlmeier, and Steven H. Zeisel, "Nutrition Education in U.S. Medical Schools: Latest Update of a National Survey," *Academic medicine: journal of the Association of American Medical Colleges* 85 (9) (2010): 1537-1542, doi: 10.1097/ACM.0b013e3181eab71b

[27] "How Food Companies Court Nutrition Educators With Junk Food, National Public Radio, May 14, 2014, http://www.npr.org/sections/thesalt/2014/05/14/312460302/how-food-companies-court-nutrition-educators-with-junk-food

[28] Dietitians for Professional Integrity, http://integritydietitians.org/

[29] "Science for Sale," Vice News, February 2016, https://news.vice.com/topic/science-for-sale

[30] "Physical Craving and Food Addiction: A Scientific Review," Philip Werdell et al., The Food Addiction Institute, 2009, http://foodaddictioninstitute.org/scientific-research/physical-craving-and-food-addiction-a-scientific-review/

[31] "Coca-Cola Presents: Happy Cycle," YouTube video, 1:39, posted by Coca-Cola, June 5, 2014, https://www.youtube.com/watch?v=N3P73agzjBg

[32] "Cognitive Dissonance," Merriam Webster, http://www.merriam-webster.com/dictionary/cognitive%20dissonance

[33] "Decision-making May Be a Surprisingly Unconscious Activity," Max-Planck-Gesellschaft, *ScienceDaily*, last modified April 15, 2008, https://www.sciencedaily.com/releases/2008/04/080414145705.htm

[34] "Zen," The Free Dictionary, http://www.thefreedictionary.com/Zen

[35] "Zen," Cambridge Dictionaries Online, http://dictionary.cambridge.org/us/dictionary/english/zen

[36] See note 3 above.

[37] Steven Covey, *The 7 Habits of Highly Effective People* (New York: Simon & Schuster, 2013, 30-31.

[38] Marion Nestle, *Soda Politics: Taking on Big Soda (and Winning)* (Oxford: Oxford University Press, 2015), 351.

[39] "Flavor enhancers, coloring agents & preservatives – Food additives demystified," *Food Democracy* (blog), October 16, 2007, https://fooddemocracy.wordpress.com/2007/10/16/food-additives-demystified/

[40] "Why 80 Percent of People Worldwide Will Soon... Stop Eating Wheat," Natasha Longo, March 30, 2012, http://www.bibliotecapleyades.net/ciencia/ciencia_geneticfood74.htm

[41] "Grains and Starchy Vegetables," American Diabetes Association, last modified February 19, 2014, http://www.diabetes.org/food-and-fitness/food/what-can-i-eat/making-healthy-food-choices/grains-and-starchy-vegetables.html?loc=ff-slabnav

[42] "FDA Limits Claims About Whole Grains," Jane Zhang and Janet Adamy, *The Wall Street Journal*, last modified December 6, 2005, http://www.wsj.com/articles/SB113382948357314612

[43] "Casein: The Disturbing Connection Between This Dairy Protein and Your Health," Heather McClees, *One Green Planet*, October 24, 2014, http://www.onegreenplanet.org/natural-health/casein-dairy-protein-and-your-health/

[44] "CASEIN PRODUCTS," C. R. Southward, *Consumer and Applications Science Section: New Zealand Dairy Research Institute*, http://nzic.org.nz/ChemProcesses/dairy/3E.pdf

APPENDIX A

Note that some nutrients are listed more than once because they fall under multiple categories.

Vitamins:
Vitamin A, Vitamin B1(Thiamine), Vitamin B2 (Riboflavin), Vitamin B3 (Niacin), Vitamin B4 (Choline), Vitamin B5(Pantothenic Acid), Vitamin B6 (Pyridoxine), Vitamin B7 (Biotin), Vitamin B8 (Inositol), Vitamin B9 (Folic Acid), Vitamin B10 (PABA or Para-Amino Benzoic Acid), Vitamin B11 (PHGA or Pteryl-Hepta-Glutamic Acid), Vitamin B12 (Cobalamin), Vitamin C (Ascorbic Acid), Vitamin C (Ascorbinogen), Vitamin C (Rutin used by blood vessels), Vitamin C (Tyrosinase is required for strengthening the effectiveness of white blood cells), Vitamin C (Factor J used for the oxygen carrying capacity of the red blood cells), Vitamin C (Factor K), Vitamin C (Factor P required for the strength of the blood vessels), Vitamin D, Vitamin E, Vitamin F (Essential Fatty Acids Omega 3 and Omega 6 – Omega 9, is usually listed separately), Vitamin G (Also referred to as Vitamin B2 or Riboflavin), Vitamin H (Also referred to as Vitamin B7 or Biotin or Vitamin I), Vitamin I (Also is occasionally referred to as B7 or Biotin or Vitamin H), Vitamin K, Vitamin L (Lysine), Vitamin P (Bioflavonoids and Flavonoids – usually occur in the same foods as Vitamin C)

Minerals:
Aluminium, Arsenic, Barium, Beryllium, Boron, Bromine, Carbon, Calcium, Cerium, Caesium, Chloride, Chromium, Cobalt, Copper, Dysprosium, Erbium, Europium, Gadolinium, Gallium, Germanium, Gold, Hafnium, Holmium, Hydrogen, Iodine, Iron, Lanthanum, Lithium, Lutetium, Magnesium, Manganese, Molybdenum, Neodymium, Niobium, Nickel, Nitrogen, Oxygen, Phosphorus, Potassium, Praseodymium, Rhenium, Rubidium, Samarium, Scandium, Selenium, Sodium, Strontium, Sulphur, Silica, Silver, Tantalum, Terbium, Thulium, Tin, Titanium, Vanadium, Ytterbium, Yttrium, Zinc, Zirconium

Amino Acids:
Valine, Lysine, Threonine, Leucine, Isoleucine, Tryptophan, Phenylalanine, Methionine, Histidine, Arginine, Taurine, Tyrosine

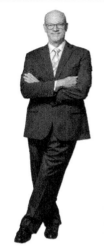
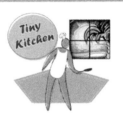
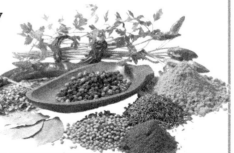

Printed in Great Britain
by Amazon

83826081R00109